National
Cancer Centre
Singapore

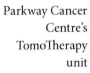

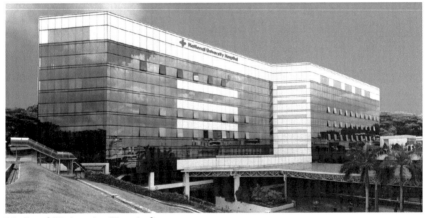

National University Hospital

Parkway Cancer
Centre's
TomoTherapy
unit

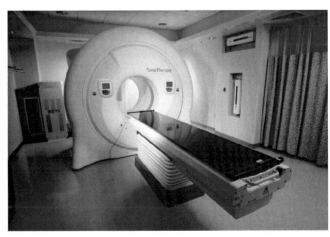

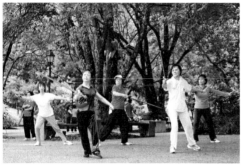

Close to the city, Singapore Botanic Gardens is home to the National Orchid and Ginger Gardens

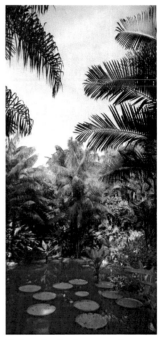

Enjoy the lushness and attractions of Singapore Botanic Gardens

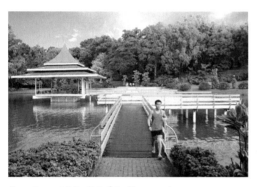

Jogging at MacRitchie Reservoir

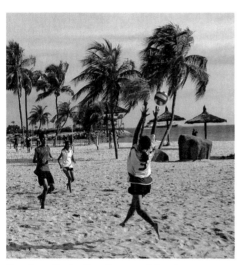

Beach volleyball at Sentosa Island

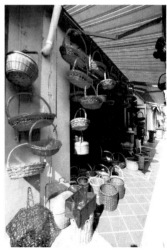

Find traditional Arab-Muslim foods and shops on Arab Street

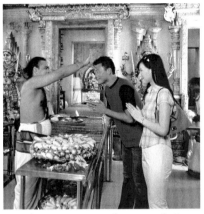

Worshippers at an Indian temple in Little India

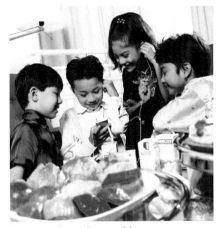

Singapore's multiracial harmony

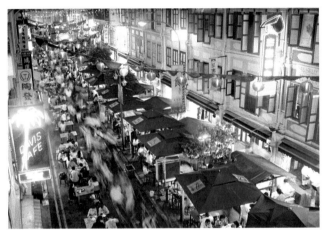

Food Street

Food Street in Chinatown

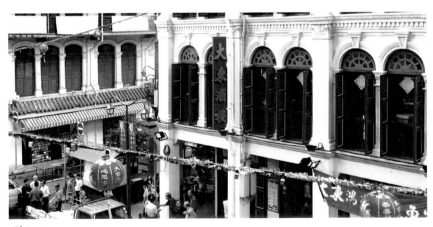

Chinatown

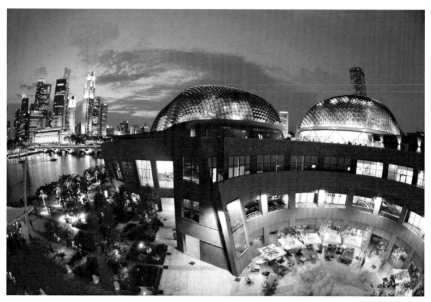

The Esplanade–Theatres on the Bay

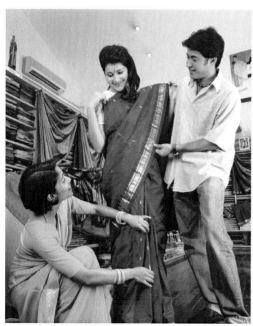

Little India is the focal point of
Singapore's Indian community

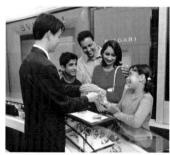

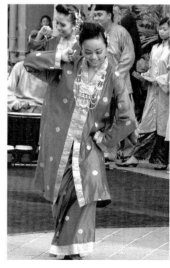

PRAISE FOR *PATIENTS BEYOND BORDERS:*

"The $20 billion-a-year global medical-tourism market finally has a guidebook of its own. With medical tourism now growing at 15 percent annually . . . this tome couldn't be more timely."

—*Travel + Leisure Magazine*

"Patients Beyond Borders tells how to plan and budget for medical care abroad and how to find the best doctors and hospitals."

—*AARP Bulletin*

"Woodman suggests a $6,000 rule: if your procedure would cost more than $6,000 in the United States, you would likely save money — possibly more than $1,000 — by traveling to a foreign hospital, including all other costs."

—NPR (National Public Radio)

"I have read and am impressed by this book."

—Arthur Frommer

"Woodman estimates that more than 150,000 Americans went abroad for medical care in 2006. Many are uninsured, self-employed or looking to defer the average $10,000 to $12,000 in insurance premiums a family of four now pays a year."

—*Forbes*

"A useful new book on this topic . . ."

—*Savvy Senior*

"I am considering elective surgery and this was a great compendium of information scattered all over the Internet."

—Amy Tupper (Sanford, NC)

"I spent a lot of time on the Internet trying to research this topic on my own and looking for certain procedures (mainly dental and cosmetic surgery). I wound up getting dental work done in Mexico at a facility reviewed in this book and am happy with my experience. I recommend this book to anyone even remotely considering foreign medical travel."

—K. Williamson (Los Lunas, NM)

"If the American healthcare system is not completely broken, it is certainly dysfunctional: 47 million people have no health coverage, and 130 million have no dental insurance. As baby boomers age into more medical problems with spotty coverage and would prefer not to deplete their retirement savings, they are looking at all available options."

—*Financial Times*

"A must-read for those considering medical tourism . . ."

—*ABC News*

"A practical guide to planning a medical trip . . ."

—*Washington Post*

Patients Beyond Borders Series™

Patients Beyond Borders
Singapore Second Edition™

Everybody's Guide to Affordable,
World-Class Medical Tourism™

Josef Woodman

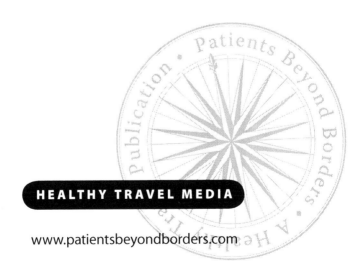

HEALTHY TRAVEL MEDIA

www.patientsbeyondborders.com

PATIENTS BEYOND BORDERS:
SINGAPORE SECOND EDITION
Everybody's Guide to Affordable, World-Class Medical Tourism

Copyright © 2008 by Josef Woodman

ISBN 13: 978-0-9791079-7-9

Cover Art and Page Design: Anne Winslow
Developmental Editing: Faith Brynie
Copyediting: Kate Johnson
Proofreading: Barbara Resch
Indexing: Madge Walls
Color Layout: Judy Orchard
Typesetting and Production: Copperline Book Services
POD Printing: Catawba Publishing, LLC
Offset Printing: C & C Offset Printers

Printed in the USA and China

Healthy Travel Media
P.O. Box 17057
Chapel Hill, NC 27516
919 370.7380
info@healthtraveler.net
www.patientsbeyondborders.com

To All the Dedicated Healthcare Workers of Singapore

Limits of Liability and Disclaimer of Warranty
Please Read Carefully

This book is intended as a reference guide, not as a medical guide or manual for self-diagnosis or self-treatment. While the intent of *Patients Beyond Borders: Singapore Second Edition* is to provide useful and informative data, neither the author nor any other party affiliated with this book renders or recommends the use of specific hospitals, clinics, professional services (including physicians and surgeons), third-party agencies, or any other source cited throughout this book.

Patients Beyond Borders: Singapore Second Edition should not be used as a substitute for advice from a medical professional. The author and publisher expressly disclaim responsibility for any adverse effects that might arise from the information found in *Patients Beyond Borders: Singapore Second Edition* or any other book, Web site, or information associated with *Patients Beyond Borders*. Readers who suspect they may have a specific medical problem should consult a physician about any suggestions made in this book.

Hospitals, clinics, or any other treatment institution cited throughout *Patients Beyond Borders: Singapore Second Edition* are responsible for all treatment provided to patients, including but not limited to surgical, medical, wellness, beauty, and all related queries, opinions, and complications. The author, publisher, editors, and all other parties affiliated with this book are not responsible for same, including any emergency, complication, or medical requirement of whatsoever nature, arising from the patient's treatment due to the patient's present or past illness, or the side effects of drugs or lack of adequate treatment. All pre-treatments, treatments, and post-treatments are the absolute responsibility of the hospital, clinic, or any other treating institution, and/or the treating physician.

ACKNOWLEDGMENTS

NEARLY FIVE YEARS and the collaboration of hundreds of patients, practitioners, providers, and institutions went into the creation of *Patients Beyond Borders* and its growing library of sister publications, including the Singapore Second Edition you are holding in your hands.

The history of this series goes back so far that it's hard to know where to begin in expressing thanks. High on the list is literary agent Peter Beren, whose energy and encouragement breathed life into my first efforts in the series. Gerald and Kathleen Hill contributed greatly to the early research. I am grateful to the dozens of gracious professionals at the Apollo Hospitals in India who helped me gain an understanding of the important health considerations behind any medical journey. Special thanks to Anil Maini, Sunita Reddy, and the consummate surgeon Vijay Bose. Also to Doug and Anne Stoda, whose courageous medical trip helped me to locate the true voice and audience for what became the First Edition of *Patients Beyond Borders*.

Today *Patients Beyond Borders* has grown to provide information on hospitals and clinics in 21 countries around the world. For helping me expand the vision as I worked on the Second Edition, I am grateful for the many insights and observations of Dan Snyder of ParkwayHealth in Singapore; Vishal Bali of Wockhardt Hospitals in India; Curtis Schroeder and Mack Banner of Bumrungrad Hospital in Thailand; James Bae of the Korea Health Industry Development Institute in South Korea; and Steven Tucker of the West Excellence Clinic in Singapore. Deep thanks also to David Boucher, Avery Comarow, Sharon Kleefield, and Karen Timmons for their pearls of wisdom, which led to new paths of research.

The original Singapore Edition of *Patients Beyond Borders* would not have been brought into the world without the vision and leadership of Dr. Jason Yap of SingaporeMedicine. Jason correctly foresaw the need for in-depth, destination-specific information, and through the original *Patients Beyond Borders: Singapore Edition*, our Country Series was born. The series now addresses half a dozen medical travel destinations and is growing steadily. I remain deeply grateful to SingaporeMedicine and the Singapore Tourism Board for their continued support and sponsorship.

Finally, a heartfelt note of appreciation to the editors, copyeditors, proofreaders, and indexers who made the Singapore Second Edition possible. Through countless sleepless nights, Felicia Tan at SingaporeMedicine worked to meet impossible deadlines and ensure the quality of data found in this book (get some rest now, Felicia!). Special thanks to our Editorial Director, Faith Brynie, and to copyeditor Kate Johnson, who polished these pages and did them proud.

Josef Woodman
Chapel Hill, NC
2008

Contents

PART TWO: SINGAPORE: MORE THAN A WORLD-CLASS HEALTH DESTINATION

PART THREE: UNIQUELY SINGAPORE

PART FOUR: RESOURCES AND REFERENCES

PREFACE TO THE
SINGAPORE SECOND EDITION

THEY SAY THAT the journey of a million miles begins with a single step. About five years ago I took such a step, embarking on a life-changing exploration of what was then termed "medical tourism." I set out to discover what overseas doctors and hospitals offer patients who can't arrange — or can't afford — elective surgeries or life-saving medical procedures in the United States, Canada, or Europe. It didn't take long to discover a relative handful of facilities offering low-cost, high-quality medical care delivered by consummate professionals in clean, comfortable, culturally friendly environments.

I've traveled more than a million miles since my journey began, and I return again and again to those countries, hospitals, physicians, and administrators who are shaping today's ever-expanding global healthcare sector. Many of them are in Singapore, a city and a nation (it's both) that boasts — according to the World Health Organization — the best healthcare system in Asia and the sixth best in the world (by comparison, the US ranks thirty-sixth.)

The first time I visited Singapore, I had already learned the country served as the hub for healthcare in Asia. Indeed, Singapore is implementing a focused national strategy to become a leading center of medical research and education for the world. These efforts are paying off, and major medical, research, and educational institutions around the globe are stepping up to collaborate. In 2005, for example, officials from Duke University Medical Center and the National University of Singapore signed an agreement to establish a new medical school in Singapore.

Another example is Biopolis, Singapore's purpose-built biomedical research complex, which opened in 2003. The facility brings together private and public research laboratories and houses the full spectrum of international research and development activities, from basic science to drug development, from genomic research to bioinformatics.

To date I've logged five trips to Singapore. Except for the long flight, traveling to Singapore is like traveling within the US. No culture shock awaits me at my destination. Singapore is an immaculate, safe, bustling, modern city where English is the language most often heard. I feel right at home there, and so do the 400,000 medical travelers who seek treatment every year in Singapore's international medical facilities.

Singapore has been receiving medical travelers for decades now, and the services that have been developed for international patients are unrivaled. Most of Singapore's international healthcare facilities run International Patient Liaison Centres that arrange everything from transplant surgery to sightseeing tours.

In my homeland of the US and in my profession, it's hard to escape all the bad news about the sorry state of the US healthcare system, its bloated bureaucracy, deteriorating hospitals, harried physicians and surgeons, rising hospital infection rates, and more. I find none of those problems when my travels take me back to Singapore. On the contrary, I find in Singapore the best of what twenty-first-century healthcare has to offer for human well-being: ultramodern facilities and advanced technical expertise mixed with a caring attitude that makes medical science all the more effective.

Whether patients, physicians, or payers—and regardless of nationality—we are all squarely in the midst of a long-overdue revolution: the globalization of healthcare. Singapore is leading the way, from its bench-to-bedside research efforts to its innovative informational and administrative structures. Those who travel the path I've taken will, I believe, choose Singapore as a preferred destination. The leadership is there. The quality is there. The service is there. What more could any medical traveler hope for?

Our editorial team and I are deeply grateful to many in Singapore for their hard work and impassioned spirit in helping to create this book. Special thanks to the vision of Jason Yap, the sleepless nights of Felicia Tan, and the support of all the friendly, hard-working colleagues at SingaporeMedicine.

Josef Woodman
November 2008

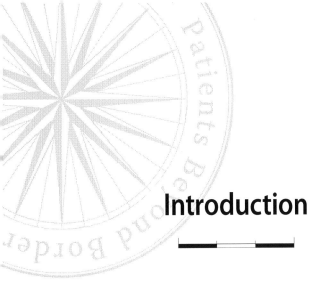

Introduction

If you're holding this copy of *Patients Beyond Borders: Singapore Second Edition* in your hands, you probably already know that you need a medical procedure, and perhaps you are considering an affordable, trustworthy alternative to care in your own country. As you can see, this is a specialty volume in the *Patients Beyond Borders* series, profiling Singapore as a healthcare destination. It is intended for those who already have (more or less) a diagnosis and already know (more or less) what treatment they need. This edition doesn't provide the breadth of general information about medical travel that you'll find in our larger book, *Patients Beyond Borders: Everybody's Guide to Affordable, World-Class Medical Travel*, now in its Second Edition. Instead, this volume offers a brief overview of the questions you need to answer before you commit to medical travel. Most of its pages are devoted to describing the best places in Singapore to find good treatment and care. It also contains information on health travel agents who can help you make arrangements for obtaining excellent medical care in Singapore at a reasonable price.

In the last two years, I have traveled to a dozen countries and visited more than 100 hospitals, talking to surgeons, healthcare administrators, and their patients. Health travelers are often pleasantly surprised at the quality of care, the prices, and the all-around good experience of their medical travel abroad. As we contemplate our options in an overburdened global healthcare environment, many of us will eventually find ourselves seeking alternatives to costly treatments — either for ourselves or for our loved ones. Healthcare consumers everywhere are in the midst of a global shift in medical services. In a few short years, big government investment, corporate partnerships, and increased media attention have spawned a new industry, medical tourism, bringing with it a host of encouraging new choices.

This new phenomenon of medical tourism — or international health travel — has recently received a good deal of wide-eyed attention. While one newspaper or blog giddily touts the fun 'n sun side of treatment abroad, another issues dire warnings about filthy hospitals, shady treatment practices, and procedures gone bad. As with most things in life, the truth lies somewhere in between. When I speak to interviewers and reporters, I try to emphasize that "medical tourism" is a misnomer. Medical travel is not a vacation. Unlike some other books on medical travel, this one focuses more on your health than on your recreational preferences. Business travelers don't consider themselves tourists; neither should you. This book will help you think about the "business" of health travel.

Patients Beyond Borders: Singapore Second Edition isn't a guide to medical diagnosis and treatment, nor does it provide medical advice on specific treatments or caregiver referrals. Your condition, diagnosis, treatment options, and travel preferences are unique, and only you — in consultation with your physician and loved ones — can determine the best course of action. Should you decide to travel abroad for treatment, we provide a wealth of resources and tools to help you become an informed medical traveler, so you can have the best possible travel experience and treatment your money can buy.

My research, including countless interviews, has convinced me that with diligence, perseverance, and good information, patients considering traveling to Singapore or other countries for treatment indeed have legitimate, safe choices, not to mention an opportunity to save thousands of dollars over the same treatment in their home country. Hundreds of patients who have returned from successful treatment overseas provide overwhelmingly positive feedback. They have persuaded me to write this series of impartial, scrutinizing guides to treatment options abroad.

Why Cross Borders for Medical Care?

Cost savings. Depending upon the country and type of treatment, uninsured and underinsured patients as well as those seeking elective care can save 15–85 percent of the cost of treatment in their home country. For example, a knee surgery that costs $43,000 in the US may cost (depending on the doctors and facilities) US$15,000 in Singapore, including your hospital stay.

Better quality care. Veteran health travelers know that facilities, instrumentation, and customer service in treatment centers abroad often equal or exceed those found in their own country.

Excluded treatments. Many people don't have health insurance. Even if you do, your policy may exclude a variety of conditions and treatments. You, the policyholder, must pay these expenses out-of-pocket.

Specialty treatments. Some procedures not available in your home country are available abroad. Some procedures that are widely practiced in certain parts of the world have not yet been approved in others, or they have been approved so recently that their availability remains spotty.

Shorter waiting periods. For decades, thousands of Canadian and British subscribers to universal, "free" healthcare plans have endured waits as long as two years for established procedures. Patients living in other countries with socialized medicine are beginning to experience longer waits as well. Some patients figure it's better to pay out-of-pocket to get out of pain or to halt a deteriorating condition than to suffer the anxiety and frustration of waiting for a far-future appointment and other medical uncertainties.

More "inpatient-friendly." Health insurance companies apply significant pressure on hospitals to move patients out of those costly beds as quickly as possible, sometimes before they are ready. As medical travelers to Singapore prepare for their journey back home, care is taken to ensure that they are discharged only at the appropriate time and no sooner. Furthermore, staff-to-patient ratios are usually higher abroad, while hospital-borne infection rates are often lower.

The lure of the new and different. Although traveling abroad for medical care can often be challenging, many patients welcome the chance to blaze a trail, and they find the creature comforts often offered abroad to be a welcome relief from the sterile, impersonal hospital environments so frequently encountered at home.

Safety and Security

The overriding concern of many patients new to global health travel is safety. That's understandable. Stories of wars, terrorist plots, roadside bombings, subway gassings, mad snipers, and military coups dominate the news. Obviously, we live in a troubled world. Yet, this fact remains: of the more than 3 million patients who traveled overseas for medical treatment in the last five years, we know of no individual who has died as a result of violence or hostility. In truth, most health travelers are usually quite sheltered. They're chauffeured from the airport to the hospital or hotel, personally driven to consultations, given their meals in their rooms, and chauffeured back to the airport when it's time to go home. US citizens who are concerned about traveling abroad can check the US Department of State's travel advisories at http://travel.state.gov/travel/cis_pa_tw/tw/tw_1764.html. Similar information services are available in other countries.

How to Use This Book

Before you dive into Part Two, please review the checklists and sidebars in **Part One, "Reminders for the Savvy, Informed Medical Traveler."** A shortened version of the more complete information in the first Singapore Edition of *Patients Beyond Borders,* it gives you some of the tools you'll need to do your research and make an informed decision. You'll find the following in Part One:

Chapter One: Dos and Don'ts for the Smart Health Traveler

Chapter Two: *Patients Beyond Borders* Budget Planner

Chapter Three: Checklists for Health Travel

  Checklist 1: Should I Consult a Health Travel Planner?

  Checklist 2: How Can a Health Travel Planner Help Me?

  Checklist 3: What Do I Need to Do Ahead of Time?

  Checklist 4: What Should I Pack?

  Checklist 5: What Should I Do Just Before and During My Trip?

  Checklist 6: What Do I Do After My Procedure?

  Checklist 7: What Does My Travel Companion Need to Do?

Part Two, "Singapore: More Than a World-Class Health Destination," begins with an overview of the country's economic, political, and social structure, healthcare system, and related industries; supplies basic, practical information you'll need to plan your trip, from time zones to visas; and provides detailed profiles of Singapore's leading healthcare establishments, including contact information as well as a rundown on available services and history of care. Accommodations are also listed, along with several health travel agencies serving medical travelers to Singapore.

Part Three, "Uniquely Singapore," describes a number of the sights and experiences to be enjoyed in Singapore.

Part Four, "Resources and References," offers additional sources of travel information and helpful links, plus a glossary of commonly used medical terms.

As you work your way through decision-making and subsequent planning, remember that you're following in the footsteps of hundreds of thousands of health travelers who have made the journey before you. The vast majority have returned home successfully treated, with money to spare in their savings accounts. Still, the process — particularly in the early planning — can be daunting, frustrating, and even a little scary. Every health traveler I've interviewed experienced "the Big Fear" at one time or another. Healthcare abroad is not for everyone, and part of being a smart consumer is evaluating all the impartial data available before making an informed decision. If you accomplish that in reading *Patients Beyond Borders: Singapore Second Edition*, I've achieved my goal. Let's get started.

Reminders for the Savvy, Informed Medical Traveler

Much of the advice here in Part One is covered in greater detail in the first Singapore Edition of *Patients Beyond Borders*. Consider the following three chapters a capsule summary of essential information, sprinkled with practical advice that will help reduce the number of inevitable "gotchas" that health travelers encounter. You may want your travel companion or family members to read this section, along with the book's Introduction, so they can gain a better understanding of medical travel.

Dos and Don'ts for the Smart Health Traveler

BEFORE YOUR TRIP

✔ *Do* plan ahead.

The farther in advance you plan, the more likely you are to get the best doctors, the lowest airfares, and the best availability and rates on hotels — particularly if you'll be traveling at peak tourist season for Singapore or any other chosen destination. If possible, begin planning at least three months prior to your expected departure date. If you're concerned about having to change plans, *do* be sure to confirm cancellation policies with airlines, hotels, and travel agents.

✔ *Do* be sure about your diagnosis and treatment needs.

The more you know about the treatment you're seeking, the easier your search for a physician will be. *Do* work closely with your local doctor or medical specialist, and make sure you obtain exact recommendations — in writing, if possible. If you lack confidence in your doctor's diagnosis, seek a second opinion.

✔ *Do* research your in-country doctor thoroughly.

This is the most important step of all. When you've narrowed your search to two or three physicians, invest some time and money in personal telephone interviews, either directly with your candidate doctors or through your health travel planning agency. *Don't* be afraid to ask questions, lots of them, until you feel comfortable that you have chosen a competent physician.

✘ *Don't* rely completely on the Internet for your research.

While it's okay to use the Web for your initial research, *don't* assume that sponsored Web sites offer complete and accurate information. Cross-check your online findings against referrals, articles in leading newspapers and magazines, word of mouth, and your health travel agent.

✔ *Do* consider traveling with a companion.

Many health travelers say they wouldn't go without a close friend or family member by their side. Your travel companion can help you every step of the way. With luck, your companion may even enjoy the trip!

✔ *Do* engage a good health travel planner.

Most of the hospitals in Singapore are now served by at least one qualified health travel agent. Even the most intrepid, adventurous medical traveler will benefit from the knowledge, experience, and in-country support these professionals can bring to any health journey. *Do* thoroughly research an agent before plunking down your deposit.

✔ *Do* get it in writing.

Cost estimates, appointments, recommendations, opinions, second opinions, airline and hotel accommodations — get as much as you can in writing, and *do* be sure to take all documentation with you on the plane. Email is fine, as long as you retain a written record of your key transactions. The more you get in writing, the less chance of a misunderstanding.

✔ *Do* insist on using a language you understand.

As much as many of us would like to have a better command of another language, the time to brush up on a foreign language is most definitely *not* when negotiating medical care! Establishing comfortable, reliable communication with your key contacts is paramount to your success as a health traveler. English-speakers who select Singapore as their healthcare destination will be glad to know that English is widely spoken, as it is the nation's business language.

✘ *Don't* plan your trip too tightly.

Don't plan your trip with military precision. A missed consultation or an extra two days of recovery can mean expensive rescheduling with airlines. A good rule of thumb is to add an extra day for every five days you anticipate for consultation, treatment, and recovery.

✔ *Do* alert your bank and credit card company.

Contact your bank and credit card company (or companies) *prior to your trip*. Inform them of your travel dates, and tell them where you will be. If you plan to use a credit card for large amounts, alert the company in advance, and reconfirm your credit limits to avoid card cancellation or unexpected rejections.

✔ *Do* learn a little about your destination.

Once you've settled on Singapore as a health travel destination, spend a little time getting to know something about its history and geography. Buy or borrow a couple of travel guides. Read a local newspaper. Your hosts will appreciate your knowledge and interest.

✔ *Do* inform your local doctors before you leave.

Preserve a good working relationship with your family physician and local specialists. Although they may not particularly like your traveling overseas for medical care, most doctors will respect your decision. Your hometown healthcare providers need to know what you are doing so they can continue your care and treatment once you return.

WHILE IN SINGAPORE

✘ *Don't* be too adventurous with local cuisine.

One sure way to get your treatment off to a bad start is to enter your clinic with even a mild case of stomach upset due to a change in water or diet. Prior to treatment, avoid rich, spicy foods and exotic drinks. Bottled water may be safer for your stomach. During any inpatient stay, *don't* be afraid to ask the hospital's dietician for a menu that's easy on your digestion.

✗ *Don't* scrimp on lodging.

Unless your finances absolutely demand it, avoid hotels and other accommodations in the "budget" category. You *don't* want to end up in uncomfortable surroundings when you are recuperating from major surgery. On the other hand, you should be able to find a good hotel in a price range that suits you. Ask your hospital or health travel agent for a recommendation.

✗ *Don't* stay too far from your treatment center.

When booking hotel accommodations for you and your companion, make sure the hospital or doctor's office is nearby. Part Two provides information on accommodations in Singapore.

✗ *Don't* settle for second best in treatment options.

While you can cut corners on airfare, lodging, and transportation, always insist on the very best healthcare your money can buy. Focus on quality, not just price.

✔ *Do* befriend the staff.

Nurses, nurse's aides, paramedics, receptionists, clerks, and even maintenance people are vital members of your health team! Take the time to chat with them, learn their names, inquire about their families, and perhaps proffer a small gift. Above all, treat the staff with deference and respect. When you're ready to leave the hospital, a sincere thank-you note makes a great farewell.

GOING HOME

✘ *Don't* return home too soon.

After a long flight to a foreign land, multiple consultations with physicians and staff, and a painful and disorienting medical procedure, most folks feel ready to jump on the first flight home. That's understandable but not advisable. Your body needs time to recuperate, and your physician needs to track your recovery progress. As you plan your trip, ask your physician how much recovery time is advised for your particular treatment. Then add a few extra days, just to be safe.

✔ *Do* set aside some of your medical travel savings for a vacation.

You and your travel companion deserve it! If you're not able to take leisure time during your trip abroad, then set aside a little money for some time off after you return home, even if only for a weekend getaway.

✔ *Do* get all your paperwork before leaving the country.

Get copies of everything. No matter how eager you are to get well and get home, make sure you have full documentation on your procedure(s), treatment(s), and followup. Get receipts for everything.

ABOVE ALL, TRUST YOUR INTUITION

Your courage and good judgment have set you on the path to medical travel. Rely on your instincts. If, for example, you feel uncomfortable with your in-country consultation, switch doctors. If you get a queasy feeling about extra or uncharted costs, don't be afraid to question them. Thousands of health travelers have beaten a well-worn path abroad, using good information and common sense. You can, too! Safe travels!

Ten "Must-Ask" Questions for Your Physician Candidate

Make the following initial inquiries, either of your health travel agent or the physician(s) you're interviewing.

1. *What are your credentials? Where did you receive your medical degree? Where was your internship? What types of continuing education workshops have you attended recently?* The right international physician either has credentials posted on the Web or will be happy to email you a complete résumé.

2. *How many patients do you see each month?* Hopefully, it's more than 50 and less than 500. The physician who says "I don't know" should make you suspicious. Doctors should be in touch with their customer base and have such information readily available.

3. *To what associations do you belong?* Any worthwhile physician or surgeon is a member of at least one medical association. Your practitioner should be keeping good company with others in the field.

4. *How many patients have you treated who have had my condition?* There's safety in numbers, and you'll want to know them. Find out how many procedures your intended hospital has performed. Ask how many of *your specific treatments for your specific condition* your candidate doctor has personally conducted.

5. *What are the fees for your initial consultation?* Answers will vary, and you should compare prices to those of other physicians you interview.

6. *May I call you on your cell phone before, during, and after treatment?* Most international physicians stay in close, direct contact with their patients, and cell phones are their tools of choice.

7. *What medical and personal health records do you need to assess my condition and treatment needs?* Most physicians require at least the basics: recent notes and recommendations from consultations with your hometown physician or specialist, x-rays directly related to your condition, perhaps a medical history, and other health records. Be wary of the physician who requires no personal paperwork.

8. *Do you practice alone, or with others in a clinic or hospital?* Look for a physician who practices among a group of certified professionals with a broad range of related skills.

For surgery:

9. *Do you do the surgery yourself, or do you have assistants do the surgery?* This is one area where delegation isn't desirable. You want assurance that your procedure won't be performed by your practitioner's protégé.

10. *Are you the physician who oversees my entire treatment, including pre-surgery, surgery, prescriptions, physical therapy recommendations, and post-surgery checkups?* For larger surgical procedures, you want the designated team captain. While that's usually the surgeon, check to make sure.

CHAPTER TWO

Patients Beyond Borders
Budget Planner

As with any other trip, your health travel costs will depend largely upon your tastes, lifestyle preferences, length of stay, side trips, and pocketbook. A patient flying first-class and staying at a five-star hotel can naturally expect less of a savings than one who spends frequent-flyer miles and lodges in a modest — but perfectly satisfactory — three-star hotel.

To derive an estimate of your health travel costs and savings, we suggest you use the *"Patients Beyond Borders* Budget Planner," below. Don't feel pressured to fill in every line item in your Budget Planner. Focus on the big expenses first, such as treatment and airfare, and then fill in the remainder as your planning progresses. You probably won't use all the categories. For example, you may already have an up-to-date passport, or you may stay only at a hospital and never visit a hotel. The Budget Planner simply lists all the common health travel expenses. As you plan, fill in the blanks that apply to you, and you'll arrive at a rough estimate of your costs — and your savings. (You'll find more details in the first Singapore Edition of *Patients Beyond Borders*.)

A Few Notes on Costs

Passport and visa. US citizens who don't have a passport and are purchasing one for the first time should budget about $200 for fees, photographs, and shipping. Passport renewal in the US costs about $150. Passport and visa fees for other countries vary widely. US citizens do not need a visa to visit Singapore for a period not exceeding 90 days. Citizens of other countries should check with the appropriate government office to determine Singaporean visa requirements.

Airfare. Air transportation will likely be your biggest nontreatment cost. It pays to shop hard for bargains. If you're okay flying coach, by all means do so; business- and first-class international travel are wildly expensive. If you have a *trusted* travel agency, use it, although with caution. Most have side deals with airlines, and their commissions and fees can cut into your savings. If you're comfortable using the Internet, take advantage of one of the many discount online travel agencies, such as Orbitz (www.orbitz.com), Expedia (www.expedia.com), Travelocity (www.travelocity.com), or CheapTickets (www.cheaptickets.com). Or go to individual airlines' Web sites, where you can sometimes snag special Internet fares.

International entry and exit fees. Many countries charge fees at the airport, and they may be due on arrival, on departure, or both. It's usually best to have cash in your pocket for these fees, which sometimes change dramatically without notice. A Passenger Service Charge of SGD21 (about US$14) is usually included in the price of an airline ticket to Singapore. If not, travelers may be required to pay the fee during check-in at the airport.

Rental car. When traveling, some people feel they can't manage without a car. Yet, international car rentals are expensive, big-city parking is a hassle, and driving in a foreign country can land you in the hospital well ahead of your scheduled stay. It's often better for the health traveler to use taxis or limousines.

Other transportation. Transportation to and from the airport will probably be handled by the hospital, your health travel agent, or the hotel where you or your companion will reside. Budget for the cost of transportation to and from your local airport, as well as for in-country transportation. Taxis and buses are usually not expensive; US$200 should cover most two-week trips.

Companions. Budget for the additional airfare and meals for your travel companion and — depending on whether you'll be doubling up — lodging. Items you can usually share include local taxi rides, mobile phone, and computer and Internet services. Items you can't share include passport and visa costs, airfare, airport fees and taxes, railway fares, meals, and entertainment.

Treatment. When you are evaluating a treatment center or physician, request the cost details in writing (email is okay), including the prices for basic treatment plus ancillaries, such as anesthesia, room fees, prescriptions, nursing services, and more. Other useful questions: Are meals included in my hospital stay? Do you supply a bed for my companion? Is there an Internet connection in the room or lobby? If you're using a health travel agency, make sure your representative gets specific answers in writing to these important questions, along with a firm cost estimate for treatment and ancillary fees.

Lodging during treatment. These costs are straightforward and are largely a function of your tastes and pocketbook. Your doctor or your treatment center's staff can provide you with a list of preferred hotels nearby.

Post-treatment lodging. It's a good idea to stick around for at least a week post-treatment, because your physician will want to keep an eye on how your recovery is progressing. Many hospitals and clinics will help you arrange accommodations nearby and plan for nursing services to meet your post-treatment needs.

Meals. If you're staying in a hospital, most of your meals will probably be provided, and the food is often surprisingly good. Many hospitals offer reasonable meal plans for companions. Ask the facility or your agent about costs for hospital meals. Otherwise, budget your dining out according to taste, both for you and for your companion.

Tips. Tipping is not customary in Singapore. It is prohibited at the airport, and it is discouraged in hotels and restaurants, where a 10 percent service charge is usually included in the bill. If your bill does not include a service charge, you may consider leaving a small tip.

Leisure travel. Many health travelers plan a vacation for either before or after treatment. While this expense isn't strictly a part of your health travel budget, you may want to add the costs of vacation-related lodging, transportation, meals, and other expenses into your estimated budget.

The $6,000 Rule

A good monetary barometer of whether your medical trip is financially worthwhile is the *Patients Beyond Borders* "$6,000 Rule": If your total quote for hometown treatment (including consultations, procedures, and hospital stay) is US$6,000 or more, you'll probably save money by traveling abroad for your care. If it's less than US$6,000, you're likely better off having your treatment at home.

The application of this rule varies, of course, depending on your financial position and lifestyle preferences. For some, a small savings might offset the hassles of travel. For others who might be traveling anyway, savings considerations are fuzzier.

Will My Health Insurance Cover My Overseas Medical Expenses?

As of this writing, it's possible, but not probable. While the largest employers and healthcare insurers — not to mention ever-vocal politicians — struggle with new models of coverage, most plans do not yet cover the costs of obtaining treatment abroad. Yet, with healthcare costs threatening to literally bust some Western economies, pressures for change are mounting. Recognizing that globalization of healthcare is now a reality — and that developed countries are falling behind — insurers, employers, and hospitals are beginning to form partnerships with payers and providers abroad. By the time you read this book, large insurers may already be offering coverage (albeit limited) across borders. Check with your insurer for the latest on your coverage abroad.

Can I Sue?

For better or worse, many countries do not share the Western attitude toward personal and institutional liability. A full discussion of the reasons lies outside the scope of this book. Here's a good rule of thumb: if legal recourse is a primary concern in making your health travel decision, you probably shouldn't head abroad for medical treatment.

If, however, you experience severe complications and do not receive the followup care you think you need or deserve, then you may want to consider legal action, say attorneys Amanda Hayes and Natasha Bellroth of Global MD. "Legal recourse and remedies are generally limited abroad for patients who experience bad outcomes in foreign facilities," they say. "Moreover, a patient's ability to sue a foreign physician or facility for medical malpractice is limited by the availability of an appropriate forum in which to bring a lawsuit."

For example, say Hayes and Bellroth, assume that American patient John Smith travels to Singapore for hip replacement surgery at ABC Hospital and suffers a bad outcome caused by his surgeon's negligence. Mr. Smith has some options for pursuing a judicial remedy:

+ In order to sue ABC Hospital in the US, a US court must be able to exercise jurisdiction over ABC Hospital, a Singaporean corporation with no offices or employees in the US. US courts may only assert general or specific personal jurisdiction over a foreign entity when the foreign entity's presence or dealings where the suit is brought justify requiring the company to defend the suit there.

+ Assuming that the case proceeds in the US to judgment against ABC Hospital, Mr. Smith faces an uphill battle to enforce an American judgment in Singapore. If Mr. Smith wins a large punitive damages award from an American court, he will be disappointed to learn that punitive damages are rarely awarded outside of the US and are unlikely to be enforced (in any of the countries currently attracting American medical travelers).

+ Alternatively, Mr. Smith may try to sue ABC Hospital in Singapore, which requires that he hire a lawyer in Singapore and perhaps travel back to Singapore to attend the proceedings. Even if Mr. Smith prevails against ABC Hospital in Singapore, he will probably only be able to recover his actual damages (the provable out-of-pocket cost of harm caused by negligence, e.g., medical bills incurred for corrective surgery, and lost wages due to time away from work), as few countries award punitive damages to successful plaintiffs.

✦ Mr. Smith may seek to arbitrate his claim against ABC Hospital before an international tribunal. For example, the International Court of Arbitration of the International Chamber of Commerce may provide Mr. Smith with a viable and likely more cost-effective way to hold ABC Hospital accountable for its negligence. Generally, an agreement to arbitrate claims must have been in place before the relationship commenced. Mr. Smith should have confirmed that prior to surgery, ABC Hospital had agreed to arbitration of potential future claims and to where those proceedings would occur.

Each alternative forum presents its own unique set of challenges. There is no ideal solution that would put judicial recourse against a foreign entity on par with the remedies available against a US hospital or physician. There are, however, practical measures that Mr. Smith might have taken before he traveled to Singapore that would have helped him manage the risk in the unlikely event of a bad outcome:

✦ For example, Mr. Smith might have purchased insurance (a health travel agency should be able to point the patient to available policies) designed specifically to protect him from the financial consequences of foreseeable complications and unforeseeable medical malpractice. Such insurance could have helped

Mr. Smith eliminate the cost of legal action while compensating him up to the amount of the policy limit he purchased.

✦ In addition, had Mr. Smith paid for his procedure with a major credit card, his card company may have allowed him to recover the cost of a disappointing treatment by disputing the charges.

✦ Finally, Mr. Smith could have made sure that his health travel agency and the treating facility had a clear and reasonable protocol in place for dealing with bad outcomes and complications. Ideally, the hospital would have agreed to absorb costs associated with making Mr. Smith whole again (return flight, accommodations, and corrective procedure) and compensate him if he could not be satisfied.

Ultimately, there is no perfect way to compensate a patient — either domestically or abroad — who has suffered an imperfect outcome after a medical procedure. The good news is that informed patients can take preventive measures to protect themselves before they travel abroad for care, so they do not end up in the hands of imperfect healthcare insurance and judicial systems.

Furthermore, foreign hospitals are eager to prove that the quality of their surgeons and technical facilities rivals and even exceeds that found in Western nations. Your independent research will reveal that sophisticated foreign hospitals and governments are heavily invested in serving international patients with high-quality healthcare; they understand that the publicity associated with even one bad outcome could quickly end the growing flow of health travelers.

Patients Beyond Borders Budget Planner

Item	Cost	Comment
IN-COUNTRY		
Passport/Visa	$200.00	For passport and visa, non-expedited
Rush charges, if any:		
Treatment Estimate		
Procedure:		
Hospital room, if extra:		Often included in treatment package
Lab work, x-rays, etc.:		
Additional consultations:		
Tips/gifts for staff:	$100.00	
Other:		
Other:		
Post-Treatment		
Recuperation lodging:		Hospital room or hotel
Physical therapy:		
Prescriptions:		
Concierge services:		Optional
Other:		
Other:		
Airfare		
You:		
Your companion:		
Other travelers:		
Airport fees:		
Other:		
Other:		
In-Country Transportation		
Taxis, buses, limos:	$200.00	
Rental car:		
Other:		
Other:		

Patients Beyond Borders Budget Planner (*continued*)

Item	Cost	Comment
Room and Board		
Hotel:		
Food:		
Entertainment/sightseeing:		
Other:		
Other:		
"While You're Away" Costs		
Pet sitter/house sitter:		
Other:		
Other:		
IN-COUNTRY SUBTOTAL		
HOMETOWN		
Procedure:		
Lab work, x-rays, etc.:		
Hospital room, if extra:		
Additional consultations:		
Physical therapy:		
Prescriptions:		
Other:		
Other:		
HOMETOWN SUBTOTAL		
TOTAL SAVINGS:		Subtract In-Country Subtotal
		from Hometown Subtotal

Patients Beyond Borders Sample Budget Planner

Item	Cost	Comment
IN-COUNTRY		
Passport/Visa	$200.00	For passport and visa, non-expedited
Rush charges, if any:		
Treatment Estimate		
Procedure:	$9,000.00	
Hospital room, if extra:		Often included in treatment package
Lab work, x-rays, etc.:	$45.00	
Additional consultations:	$200.00	
Tips/gifts for staff:	$100.00	
Other:		
Other:		
Post-Treatment		
Recuperation lodging:	$1,100.00	Hospital room or hotel
Physical therapy:		
Prescriptions:	$65.00	
Concierge services:	$300.00	Optional
Other:		
Other:		
Airfare		
You:	$880.00	
Your companion:	$880.00	
Other travelers:		
Airport fees:	$14.00	
Other:		
Other:		
In-Country Transportation		
Taxis, buses, limos:	$200.00	
Rental car:		
Other:		
Other:		

Patients Beyond Borders Sample Budget Planner (*continued*)

Item	Cost	Comment
Room and Board		
Hotel:	$1,500.00	
Food:	$650.00	
Entertainment/sightseeing:	$500.00	
Other:		
Other:		
"While You're Away" Costs		
Pet sitter/house sitter:	$300.00	
Other:		
Other:		
IN-COUNTRY SUBTOTAL	$15,943.00	
HOMETOWN		
Procedure:	$55,000.00	
Lab work, x-rays, etc.:	$375.00	
Hospital room, if extra:	$4,400.00	
Additional consultations:		
Physical therapy:	$400.00	
Prescriptions:	$500.00	
Other:		
Other:		
HOMETOWN SUBTOTAL	$60,675.00	
TOTAL SAVINGS:	$44,741.00	Subtract In-Country Subtotal
		from Hometown Subtotal

Your Medical Trip May Be Tax-Deductible

What do Hainanese chicken rice, taxi rides, and treatments have in common? All these expenses may be tax-deductible as part of your health travel. Depending upon your income level and cost of treatment, some or most of your health journey can be itemized as a straight deduction from your adjusted gross income.

In brief, if you're itemizing your deductions, and if IRS-authorized medical treatment and related expenses amount to more than 7.5 percent of your adjusted gross income, you're allowed to deduct the remainder of those expenses, whether they were incurred in Toledo, Ohio, or Toledo, Spain.

For example, if your adjusted gross income is US$90,000, then any allowed medical expense over $6,750 ($90,000 × 7.5 percent) becomes a straight deduction. Suppose, for example, that your medical trip cost you a total of $14,000, including treatment, travel, lodging, and, of course, a two-week surgeon-recommended stay in a five-star beachfront recuperation resort. For that trip, you could deduct $7,250 ($14,000 − $6,750) from your adjusted gross income.

Of course, your expenses must be directly related to your treatment, and many specific items are disallowed. Examples of typical tax-deductible items include:

- Any treatment normally covered by a health insurance plan
- Transportation expenses, including air, train, boat, or car travel
- Lodging and in-treatment meals
- Recovery hotels, surgical retreats, and recuperation resorts

Be sure to save all your receipts and keep a detailed expense log, noting time, date, purpose, and amount paid. Ask for letters and other documentation from your in-country healthcare provider, particularly any recommendations made for outside lodging, special diets, and other services.

For more information, you can go straight to the source. Go to www.irs.gov, or call the IRS directly at 800 829.1040. Consult a competent tax advisor with questions or concerns.

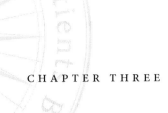

Checklists
for Health Travel

If you're like most readers of this book, you are *almost* sure that
health travel is the right choice. You have a diagnosis and you
know what medical procedure is required. You've reviewed the
costs for your procedure at home and are beginning to believe
that treatment abroad offers significant advantages — mostly
financial.

But, if you are like most patients contemplating medical care
abroad, you know you have some homework to do before you get
on a plane and head to a hospital or clinic overseas. While this
book focuses primarily on destinations for treatment in Singapore, it's a good idea to reconsider some of the questions that
apply to all health travelers — no matter what their treatment or
destination.

The seven checklists that follow will remind you of some issues
and items you might forget. Review and check off those things
that apply to your situation, and you'll increase your chances

of a safe, happy, and healthy outcome. If you desire additional information about traveling abroad for treatment, you may want to buy or borrow a copy of the first Singapore Edition of *Patients Beyond Borders,* which contains greatly expanded information for medical travelers.

CHECKLIST 1: *Should I Consult a Health Travel Planner?*

Health travel planners answer to many names: brokers, facilitators, agents, expediters. Throughout this book, we use the phrase "health travel planner" or "health travel agent" to mean any agency or representative who specializes in helping patients obtain medical treatment abroad (several are listed in Part Two of this book). Before engaging the services of a health travel agent, ask yourself these questions:

WHETHER TO USE A HEALTH TRAVEL PLANNER	Yes	No	Not Sure	Notes to Myself
Will a health travel planner save me time?				
Am I willing to pay for the convenience of a health travel planner's services?				
Will I feel more confident about health travel if I use the services of an agency?				
Does the agent I'm considering have the knowledge and experience I need?				
Does this planner have a track record of successful service to the health traveler?				
Does this agent speak my language well enough for us to converse comfortably?				
Can I get at least two recommendations or letters of reference from former clients of this agency? Have I checked these references?				
Can I get at least two recommendations or letters of reference from treatment centers that work with this agency?				

(continued)

WHETHER TO USE A HEALTH TRAVEL PLANNER	Yes	No	Not Sure	Notes to Myself
Can this agency give me complete information about possible destinations and options for my procedure?				
Will this agent put me in touch with one or more treatment centers and physicians?				
Will this agent work collaboratively to help me choose the best treatment option?				
Is this agent responsive to my questions and concerns?				
Does the service package this agent is offering meet my needs?				
Does this agent have longstanding affiliations with in-country treatment centers and practitioners?				
Has this planner negotiated better-than-retail rates with hospitals, clinics, physicians, hotels, and (perhaps) airlines?				
Can this agent save me money on other in-country costs, such as airport pickup and dropoff or transportation to my clinic?				
Can this agent offer personal assistance and support in my destination country?				
Is this planner willing to work within the constraints of my budget?				
Do I know (and have in writing) the exact costs for this agency's services?				
Do I have a suitable contract or letter of agreement with this agency?				
Do I feel comfortable with this agency? Have we built a sense of trust?				

When *Not* to Use a Health Travel Planner

Don't use an agent who does not promptly answer your initial requests for information, does not reasonably follow through on commitments, or does not treat you well in any way. Difficulty deciphering an agent's communications is a red flag, too. If a trusted friend or other reliable source has referred you to a specific clinic and physician, then half the work is already done, and you may want to forgo an agent's services, particularly if the hospital or clinic provides similar services (for instance, through its international patients center).

Paying for a Health Travel Planner's Services

Some planners offer "all-in-one" package deals, which are fine. However, at tax time, you may need to show your itemized cost breakdown, including treatment, lodging, meals, transportation, and health travel agent fees. Spreadsheets are universal these days. Ask your planner to give you a detailed expense log.

Costs and payments are usually handled in one of three ways:

Membership, upfront fee required. This arrangement requires the patient to pay a nonrefundable membership fee (often in the US$50–300 range) before any services are rendered. The membership fee is usually folded into the package price if you engage that agent.

Package, advance deposit required. In this arrangement, an agent first provides enough information to get you well along your path: data on specific treatment centers and physicians, advice on medical records and in-country procedures, and perhaps even a telephone consultation with your candidate physician or surgeon. At that point, if you decide to engage the agent, you'll be asked to submit a deposit, perhaps 25–50 percent of the entire package price. Another payment is due prior to treatment, and the remainder is payable when you leave the hospital or clinic.

Pay as you go, direct to third parties. A handful of planners act more as referral services than as full-blown brokers, providing information about hospitals and physicians, airfares, and vacation opportunities, without doing much of the real legwork. They usually charge you a commission or set fee on any service you engage.

If you're dealing with a reputable agent, all these fee structures get you to much the same place. Beware, however, of agents asking for 100 percent up front. You should see evidence of performance, communicate with all the parties personally (via telephone or email), and know that your hard-earned money is going where it should.

Although a deposit of up to 50 percent of the total package cost is usually required, you should reserve at least 25 percent of the total bill for final payment. In other words, as with most other services, don't pay the entire bill until you're satisfied and all the services you were promised have been provided. Most planners accept credit cards, but before you use yours, ask your agent about any surcharges associated with credit card payments.

CHECKLIST 2: *How Can a Health Travel Planner Help Me?*

Of all the services a health travel planner offers, the most important are related to your treatment. Start your dialogue by asking the fundamental questions: Do you know the best doctors? Have you met personally with your preferred physicians and visited their clinics? Can you give me their credentials and background information? What about accommodations? Do you provide transportation to and from the airport? To and from the treatment center? If an agent is knowledgeable and capable with these details, the rest of the planning usually takes care of itself.

DOES MY HEALTH TRAVEL PLANNER PROVIDE THIS SERVICE?	Yes	No	Not Sure	Notes to Myself
Treatment options from which to choose destination countries, hospitals, and physicians best equipped to meet my needs				
Information on hospital accreditation and physicians' credentials, board affiliations, number of surgeries performed, association memberships, and ongoing training				
Appointment scheduling and confirmations for tests, consultations, and treatments				
Teleconsultation with physicians or surgeons to review my medical history and discuss my procedure				
Transfer of medical records, including history, x-rays, test results, recommendations, and other documentation				
Travel arrangements, including airline and hotel reservations, tickets, and confirmations; also including local in-country transportation				
Visa or passport facilitation				
Onsite pre-treatment assistance, including a local representative to accompany me to appointments, expedite hospital admission, arrange local transportation, and assist with my hospital discharge				
Recovery arrangements, including local transportation, lodging, meals, and any nursing services required during recovery				

(continued)

DOES MY HEALTH TRAVEL PLANNER PROVIDE THIS SERVICE?	Yes	No	Not Sure	Notes to Myself
Amenity arrangements, including "concierge services," such as take-out food from restaurants, tickets for events, and dry-cleaning and laundry services				
Communications arrangements, including cell phone, telephone, and Internet services				
Leisure or vacation planning (if desired)				
Aftercare and followup once I've returned home, including post-treatment liaison for information retrieval and making arrangements for a return trip should complications arise				

CHECKLIST 3: *What Do I Need to Do Ahead of Time?*

Although each journey varies according to the traveler's preferences and pocketbook, good planning is essential to the success of any trip. That goes double for the medical traveler. This checklist covers some of the planning you'll need to do to become a fully prepared and informed global patient.

Why should you plan at least three months in advance?

- **The best overseas physicians are also the busiest.** If you want the most qualified doctor and the best care your global patient money can buy, give the doctors and treatment centers you select plenty of time to work you into their calendars.

- **The lowest international airfares go to those who book early.** Booking at least 60 days prior to treatment avoids the unhappy upward spiral of air travel costs. If you're planning to redeem frequent-flyer miles, try to book at least 90 days in advance.

- **Peak seasons can snarl the best-laid plans.** International tourism is on the rise, and you can encounter problems if you want or need to travel during the busy tourist season.

- **Everything takes longer than you think it will.** It's simply a fact of life.

For Big Surgeries, Think Big

Y ou want to be certain you're getting the best. For big surgeries, I advise heading to the big hospitals that have performed large numbers of *exactly* your kind of procedure, with the accreditation and success ratios to prove it. A JCI-accredited hospital carries the necessary staff, medical talent, administrative infrastructure, state-of-the-art instrumentation, and institutional followup you need.

Singapore has a large number of JCI-accredited hospitals, including the following:

National Healthcare Group
Institute of Mental Health/Woodbridge Hospital
Johns Hopkins Singapore International Medical Centre
National University Hospital
Tan Tock Seng Hospital
Alexandra Hospital
National Skin Centre

Parkway Group Healthcare (ParkwayHealth)
Gleneagles Hospital
Mount Elizabeth Hospital
East Shore Hospital

Singapore Health Services (SingHealth)
Changi General Hospital
KK Women's and Children's Hospital
Singapore General Hospital
National Heart Centre Singapore

(**Note:** For more information on JCI, the Joint Commission International, see "The What and Why of JCI," below. See also "Alternatives to JCI.")

Be sure to ask about success and morbidity rates *for your particular procedure* and find out how they compare with those at home. If you are having surgery, ask your surgeon how many surgeries *of exactly your procedure* he or she has performed in the past two years. While there are no set standards, fewer than ten is not so good. More than 50 is much better.

HAVE I COMPLETED THESE PLANNING STEPS?	Yes	No	Notes to Myself
Engaged the services of a health travel planner (if desired — see Checklists 1 and 2)			
Obtained a second opinion — or a third if necessary — on diagnosis and treatment options			
Considered a range of treatment options and discussed each option with potential providers			
Reviewed the various hospitals, clinics, specialties, and treatments available to select an appropriate destination (see Part Two)			
Chosen a reliable, fun travel companion			
Obtained and reviewed the professional credentials of two or more physicians or surgeons (see "Ten 'Must-Ask' Questions for Your Physician Candidate" in Chapter One)			
Selected the best physician or surgeon for the treatment I need			
Researched the history and accreditation of the hospital or clinic (see "The What and Why of JCI" and "Alternatives to JCI," below)			
Checked for the affiliations and partnerships of the hospital or clinic			
Learned about the number of surgeries performed in the hospital or clinic (generally, the more the better)			
Learned about success rates (these are usually calculated as a ratio of successful operations to overall number of operations performed)			
Gathered and sent all medical records and diagnostic information that my physician or surgeon needs to plan my treatment			
Prearranged travel, accommodations, recovery, and leisure activities (if desired)			
Prearranged amenities, such as concierge services in-country or wheelchair services on the return trip			
Packed the essentials (see Checklist 4)			
Double-checked everything — then checked again			

The What and Why of JCI

When you walk into a hospital or clinic in the US and many other Western countries, chances are good it's accredited, meaning that it's in compliance with standards and "good practices" set by an independent accreditation agency. In the US, by far the largest and most respected accreditation agency is the Joint Commission. The commission casts a wide net of evaluation for hospitals, clinics, home healthcare, ambulatory services, and a host of other healthcare facilities and services throughout the US.

Responding to a global demand for accreditation standards, in 1999 the Joint Commission launched its international affiliate accreditation agency, the Joint Commission International (JCI). In order to be accredited, an international healthcare provider must meet the rigorous standards set forth by JCI.

Although JCI accreditation is not essential, it's an important new benchmark and the only medically oriented seal of approval for international hospitals and clinics. Learning that your treatment center is JCI-approved lends a comfort to the process, and the remainder of your searching and checking need not be as rigorous. That said, many excellent hospitals, while not JCI-approved, have received local accreditation at the same levels as the world's best treatment centers.

JCI's Web site carries far more information than you'll ever want to explore on accreditation standards and procedures. To view JCI's current roster of accredited hospitals abroad, go to www.jointcommissioninternational.com; in the left column, click "JCI Accredited Organizations."

Alternatives to JCI

When researching hospitals and clinics abroad, you'll often come across the phrase "ISO-accredited." Based in Geneva, Switzerland, the International Organization for Standardization (ISO) is a 157-country network of national standards institutes that approves and accredits a wide range of product and service sectors worldwide, including hospitals and clinics. ISO mostly oversees facilities and administration, not healthcare procedures, practices, or methods. Thus, while ISO accreditation is good to see, it's of limited value in terms of your treatment.

Other organizations around the world set standards and accredit hospitals, and some may be as careful in their procedures and protocols as JCI — *or not*. JCI is the only organization that demands the equivalent of US healthcare standards in hospitals accredited abroad. Other organizations that accredit in non-JCI countries include the International Society for Quality in Healthcare, the Australian Council of Healthcare Standards, the Canadian Council on Health Services Accreditation, the Irish Health Services Accreditation Board, the Council for Health Services Accreditation of Southern Africa, the Japan Council for Quality in Health Care, and the Egyptian Health Care Accreditation Organization. If you are considering a hospital accredited by one of these organizations, it pays to investigate the criteria applied to the accreditation and determine to your own satisfaction that the standards are sufficient and appropriate to your needs.

CHECKLIST 4: *What Should I Pack?*

You've likely heard the cardinal rule of international travel: pack light. Less to carry means less to lose. Don't worry if you leave behind some basic item, such as shampoo or a comb, as you can always pick it up at your destination. That said, this checklist covers the items you absolutely, positively shouldn't forget — and make sure to carry these things in your carry-on bag. A prescription or passport lost in checked luggage could spell disaster.

IS THIS ITEM PACKED IN MY CARRY-ON BAG?	Yes	No	Notes to Myself
Passport			
Visa (if required)			
Travel itinerary			
Airline tickets or eticket confirmations			
Driver's license or valid picture ID (in addition to passport)			
Health insurance card(s) or policy			
ATM card or traveler's checks			
Credit card(s)			
Enough cash for airport fees and local transportation on arrival			
Immunization record			
Prescription medications			
Hard-to-find over-the-counter drugs			
Medical records, current x-rays, consultations, and treatment notes			
All financial agreements and hard copies of email correspondence			
Phone and fax numbers, mailing addresses, and email addresses of people I need or want to contact in-country			
Phone and fax numbers, mailing addresses, and email addresses of people I need or want to contact back home			
Travel journal for notes, expense records, and receipts			

CHECKLIST 5: *What Should I Do Just Before and During My Trip?*

Now that you've made appointments with one or more physicians, booked your airfare and hotel, and arranged transportation, the hard part is behind you — except, of course, for the treatment itself. You'll find that once you arrive in-country, you will be greeted graciously with help and support from hotel and hospital staff, your health travel agent, and sometimes even a friendly bystander.

If you haven't done much international traveling prior to this health journey, keep in mind that you don't need to be a seasoned travel veteran to have a successful trip. Getting things done cooperatively and efficiently will help you and your companion preserve your physical *and* mental health. Knowing a little something about the culture, history, geography, and language of your host country will buy you boatloads of goodwill and appreciation.

Tick off the items on this checklist to make sure you stay safe, happy, and well before and during your trip.

PREPARATIONS FOR MY TRIP	Yes	No	Not Sure	Notes to Myself
Have I read (or at least skimmed) a travel book or some brochures about the history, culture, and government of my destination country?				
Have I learned a few phrases, such as "please" and "thank you," in the local language?				
Have I studied a map of the city or country I'm visiting?				
Do I know what the local currency is, what the exchange rate is, and how I can pay for my needs in my destination country?				
Do I know the rules about the amount of cash I can carry into and out of my destination country?				
Have I found out what extra fees I will be charged for using my credit cards or ATM cards overseas?				
If I want to use traveler's checks, am I sure that my service providers will accept them? (Some don't.)				

(continued)

PREPARATIONS FOR MY TRIP	Yes	No	Not Sure	Notes to Myself
Am I leaving my valuables at home?				
If I must carry valuables, am I sure that a hotel safe or a safe deposit box will be available to me?				
Am I prepared to drink only bottled water and eat only cooked foods? (This is a wise precaution for both the health traveler and the companion.)				
Have I packed a sanitizer for cleaning my hands everywhere I travel?				
Have I packed comfortable clothes that are sensitive to local customs of dress? (For example, you may be expected to cover your head, arms, or legs in some countries.)				
Have I made arrangements for telephone and email service that will allow me to stay in touch with friends and relatives back home? With service providers in-country?				
Am I sure my cell phone will work overseas?				
Have I informed my doctor of all my pre-existing health conditions, such as diabetes, heart disease, ulcers, and others?				
Have I informed my physician about all prescription and over-the-counter drugs I am taking, including vitamins, minerals, and herbal supplements?				
Am I following my doctor's instructions pre-treatment, such as going off certain drugs, losing weight, or avoiding alcohol?				

Continuity of Care — Critical to Success

Continuity of care can be a challenge for patients who travel for medical procedures, say Steven Gerst, MD, and John Linss of MedicaView International (www.medicaview.com). Typically, the patient's primary physician diagnoses the condition and then suggests treatment. When the patient chooses to travel to another location or country to receive the treatment, the primary physician is too often left out of the process.

Similarly — and amazingly enough — many traveling patients engage a facility to perform a procedure without speaking directly to the surgeon before arriving. The patient and the hospital's international patient services coordinator may use email for preliminary communications. There may also be a telephone call or two with the coordinator. But the surgeon may not become actively involved until the patient arrives at the facility.

Too many patients make the assumption that a diagnosis is the "end of the story" and that contact with the coordinator is all that is required. *They could not be more wrong!*

Establish Communication!

If you're the patient, insist on speaking to the surgeon who will perform the procedure *before* you schedule your travel. You may communicate via teleconference, videoconference, or voice over Internet protocol (VOIP).

It is equally important that you establish communication between your primary (local) doctor and your overseas surgeon, so followup care is prearranged. Because of time zone and language differences, this advance planning may be difficult, but it is essential. Complications and misunderstandings can arise if your doctors are not communicating properly. For example, after a knee replacement or a kidney transplant, many concerns and complications can arise during the long recuperation period. Lack of communication can result in unnecessary hardships and potential returns to surgery.

Once you choose to go outside your physician's primary network, few mechanisms currently exist to encourage and facilitate ongoing consultations. *You must establish your own.* Critical information about your case can be lost if you don't. *Be proactive!* Here and abroad, it is usually up to you, the patient, to keep the dialogue going between your physicians.

Persistence is important, and the time-delayed effectiveness of email comes in handy — once you get the doctors in the habit of emailing each other and you. A secure online collaboration tool is even better, because it can keep all communications in one place and available to all participants at any time.

Have Your Most Current Medical Records

Once you have established contact with an overseas doctor (or surgeon) and facility, provide them with your most current medical records. If you have a chronic condition and you've finally said "enough," your medical records may be a year or more old. If they are, visit your physician to obtain new laboratory tests, x-rays, MRI or CT scans — whatever your overseas provider needs.

Medical records can be transmitted in two ways: you can send paper copies or disks by postal service, or you can send electronic documents via a secure online service. An online service is preferable for several reasons. First, it gets the records in the hands of the surgeon more quickly. Second, it creates a secure repository that can be accessed by both your hometown and overseas doctors. Third and most important, digital records create a foundation for aftercare collaboration.

Collaboration Between Your Local Doctor and Your Overseas Surgeon

Transferring your medical records may get your local doctor communicating with your overseas doctor for the first time. This communication can be achieved though email, telephone, or a private group set-up in an online environment specifically designed for that purpose. Often such an environment is part of an online repository system that provides a secure place for collaboration between the doctors via protected blog, chat, email, and VOIP.

The next collaboration between doctors should occur after surgery. The surgeon should notify your hometown physician, preferably through an online system, of the details of the surgery and the aftercare protocol.

Once you return home and are again under the care of your local physician, collaboration and consultation should continue. This collaboration should carry on until you are released from care with a clean bill of health.

Complete Documentation

Frequently, when such a repository system is not utilized, patients return home lacking the complete documentation their local physician needs to oversee ongoing care. The absence of information compromises the physician's effectiveness and threatens the patient's health.

Be sure to ask the surgical facility if access is available to an electronic system of medical record–sharing and physician collaboration. If not, request that your overseas healthcare providers subscribe to one to ensure that you can keep your local physician informed.

At a minimum, make sure your in-country facility provides you with complete records when you return home. Also make sure you keep your hometown physician involved from the first day. Good continuity of care is essential for a successful outcome.

Remember, as a patient, you need to take responsibility for the quality and consistency of the care you receive. If you don't, no one else will!

CHECKLIST 6: *What Do I Do After My Procedure?*

You've been out of surgery for two days, you hurt all over, your digestive system is acting up, and you're running a fever. Have you somehow contracted an antibiotic-resistant staph infection? Coping with post-surgery discomfort is difficult enough when you're close to home. Lying for long hours in a hospital bed, far away from family — that's often the darkest time for a health traveler.

Knowledge is the best antidote to needless worry. As with pre-surgery preparation, ask lots of questions about post-surgery discomforts *before* heading into the operating room. Be sure to ask doctors and nurses about what kinds of discomforts to expect following your specific procedure.

If your discomfort or pain becomes acute, bleeding is persistent, or you suspect a growing infection, you may be experiencing a complication that is more serious than mere discomfort and requires immediate attention. Contact your physician without delay.

This checklist will help you make the most of your post-treatment period and know when it's appropriate to seek medical assistance.

POST-PROCEDURE PREPARATIONS AND FOLLOWUP	Yes	No	Not Sure	Notes to Myself
Have I received all my doctor's instructions for my post-treatment care and recovery? Do I understand them all?				
Am I following all of my physician's instructions *to the letter?*				
Do I know what post-treatment signs and symptoms are normal?				
Do I know what post-treatment signs and symptoms indicate a need for prompt medical attention? (See "Post-Treatment: Normal Discomfort or Something More Complicated?" below.)				
Do I have copies of all my medical records and treatment records, including x-rays, photographs, blood test results, prescriptions, and others?				
Do I have itemized receipts for all the bills I have paid?				
Do I have itemized bills for all the costs I have not yet paid?				
Do I have completed insurance claim forms (if applicable)?				
Have I allotted ample time for recovery?				
Do I know how to prevent blood clots in the legs after surgery and on the airplane? (See "Caution: Blood Clots in the Veins," below.)				
Do I know what followup treatment I will need when I return home, including physical therapy?				
Have I let my family know what help I will need after I return home?				
Have I checked in with my local doctor to share information about the procedure I had and my post-treatment care needs?				
Am I staying mentally, physically, and socially active following my procedure?				

Post-Treatment: Normal Discomfort or Something More Complicated?

Prior to your surgery, your doctor should thoroughly explain the procedure and tell you about discomforts you can expect after being wheeled out of the operating unit. Discomforts differ from complications. Discomforts are predictable and unthreatening. Complications, while rarely life-threatening, are more serious and may require medical attention. These are some common discomforts you can expect following surgery:

+ minor local pain and general achiness

+ swelling

+ puffiness

+ bruising, swelling, and minor bleeding around the incision

+ headaches (side effect of anesthesia)

+ urinary retention or difficulty urinating (side effect of anesthesia and catheters)

+ nausea and vomiting, dry mouth, temporary memory loss, lingering tiredness (all common side effects of anesthesia)

+ hunger and undernutrition

Most surgically induced discomforts recede or disappear altogether during the first few days after treatment, as the body and spirit return to normal. Be sure, however, to report discomforts that persist or become more pronounced, as they might be early warning signs of more serious complications.

Complications vary according to each surgery, and you should make sure you're aware of the more common ones. Complications are scary, and many doctors would rather not go into morbid detail about them unless pressed. Complications are rare; most arise in less than 5 percent of all cases — and generally among patients who are aged or infirm in the first place. So while it's wise to be informed and vigilant, there's no need to worry yourself sick anticipating the worst. Common symptoms of complications include the following:

✦ infection, increased pain, or swelling around the incision

✦ abnormal bleeding around the incision

✦ sudden or unexplained high fever

✦ extreme chest pain or shortness of breath

✦ extreme headache

✦ extreme difficulty urinating

If you experience any of those symptoms, call your physician immediately.

Caution: Blood Clots in the Veins

Recent surgery and the immobility of long flights increase the risk of deep vein thrombosis (DVT), a term that describes the formation of a clot, or thrombus, in one of the deep veins, usually in the lower leg. The symptoms of DVT may include pain and redness of the skin over a vein, or swelling and tenderness in the ankle, foot, or thigh. More serious symptoms include chest pain and shortness of breath.

You can take preventive steps to reduce your risk of DVT, such as wearing compression stockings and moving about frequently when on planes and trains. Ask your doctor about how soon after surgery you can undertake a long, sedentary trip.

OTHER WAYS TO REDUCE RISKS

Before you travel:

- Stop smoking.
- Lose weight if you need to.
- Get enough exercise to be at least minimally fit before your surgery and your travel.
- Discuss stopping birth control pills and hormone replacement therapy with your doctor.
- Travel on an airline that provides sufficient leg room.
- Wear loose clothing.
- Reserve an aisle seat on the airplane so you can get up and move around easily.
- Ask your surgeon about using a pneumatic compression device during and after surgery.
- Before your flight home, ask your surgeon if you need an anticoagulant.
- Walk briskly for at least half an hour before takeoff.

On the plane:

- Don't stow your carry-on luggage under your seat if it restricts your movement.
- Flex your calves and rotate your ankles every 20–30 minutes.
- Walk up and down the aisle every two hours or more frequently.
- Sleep only for short periods.
- Do not take sleeping pills.
- Drink lots of water to avoid dehydration.
- Avoid alcohol, caffeine, and diet soda.
- Wear elastic flight socks or support stockings.
- Don't let your stockings or clothing roll up or constrict your legs.
- Take deep breaths frequently throughout your flight.

The Straight Dope on Pharmaceuticals

- *True or false:* When traveling, it's okay to bring small amounts of prescription drugs back into your home country.
- *True or false:* It's legal to order prescriptions from reputable online pharmacies outside your home country.

Believe it or not — for many Western countries — the answer is false on both counts, though with some favorable caveats.

Many international travelers like to purchase their favorite prescription medications less expensively while abroad. While it's *technically* illegal in the US and some other countries, consumer activists have turned the issue into a political hot potato.

Consequently, at this writing, customs inspectors are often reluctant to bust granny with her two vials of benazepril, and in most instances they turn a blind eye to folks entering the country with prescription medications purchased abroad. Thus, it's become a gray area, with customs inspectors empowered to use "general discretion" when prescription drugs are found. Most often, the offending pharmaceuticals are simply confiscated, and the traveler must decide whether it's worth all the red tape required to petition for their return.

The overwhelming majority of tourists carrying pharmaceuticals purchased abroad enter the country with no trouble, usually unnoticed. The best advice is to use common sense. You're far less likely to be hassled carrying a single prescription of amoxicillin than if your suitcase is bursting with enough tramadol to supply the streets of Los Angeles for a year. And as always, if you're carrying drugs that are illegal — prescription or otherwise — you may be subject to arrest, as well as seizure of your medications.

Similarly, it's *technically* illegal in the US and some other countries to purchase any pharmaceutical of any kind from any mail-order pharmacy outside the country. Again, highly vocal activists have prevailed politically in the US and elsewhere, and only a small fraction of prescription drugs purchased from foreign countries is seized. In those cases, the pharmacies often double-ship the order, so the buyer usually doesn't even know the purchase was interrupted.

Again, until the laws change, you're advised to use good judgment. Purchase only from reputable pharmacies, using legitimate prescriptions from your physician. And anticipate the outside chance you'll be among the few every year inconvenienced by border seizures of prescription drugs.

It's perfectly legal to purchase prescriptions online from authorized mail-order pharmacies inside your home country.

For specifics about bringing controlled substances into the US, call 202 307.2414. US citizens can obtain additional information about traveling with medication from any FDA office or by writing to the US Food and Drug Administration, Division of Import Operations and Policy, Room 12-8 (HFC-170), 5600 Fishers Lane, Rockville, MD 20857. For further information on prescription drug rules and regulations, US citizens can contact the FDA's Center for Drugs at 888 INFO.FDA or visit www.fda.gov/cder. Citizens of other countries are encouraged to contact the appropriate government office for full rules and regulations.

CHECKLIST 7: *What Does My Travel Companion Need to Do?*

A person who accompanies a health traveler gives a great gift. Here are some questions for potential companions to answer before they commit themselves to accompanying a health traveler abroad.

TRAVEL COMPANION'S CONSIDERATIONS	Yes	No	Not Sure	Notes to Myself
Am I sure I want to go? Am I sure I'm up to the task? (If you hesitate in answering either question, you may want to reconsider.)				
Am I willing and able to take responsibility for handling details, such as visas and passports?				
Do I feel comfortable acting as an advocate for the health traveler at times when he or she may need assistance?				
Have we agreed on the costs of the trip and who is responsible for paying what?				
Do I feel sufficiently confident about handling experiences and challenges in a foreign country, such as getting through airports, arranging for taxis, or finding addresses?				
Do the health traveler and I communicate well enough to identify problems and solve them together amicably?				
Am I prepared to listen to and record doctor's instructions and provide reminders for the health traveler when needed?				
Can I help the health traveler stay in touch with family, friends, and healthcare providers back home?				
Have I allowed for "down time" and time for myself during the medical travel?				
Do I have the patience to help the health traveler through what might be a long and difficult recovery period, both abroad and back home?				

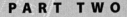

SINGAPORE:
More Than a World-Class
Health Destination

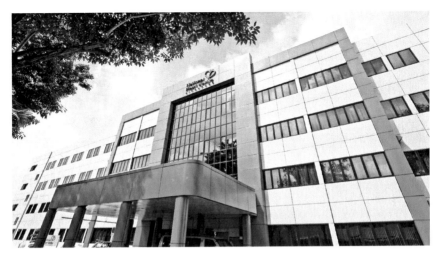

National Heart Centre

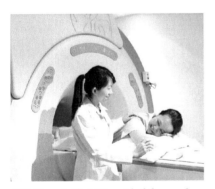

KK Hospital's MR-guided focused
ultrasound unit

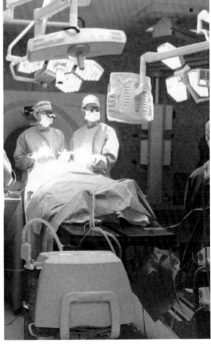

Intra-operative image-guided
navigation at National Neuroscience
Institute

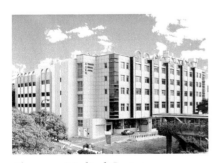

Thomson Medical Centre

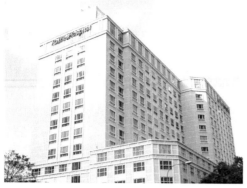
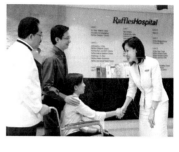

Located in the heart of Singapore, Raffles Hospital offers an array of specialist services combined with advanced medical technology in luxurious surroundings

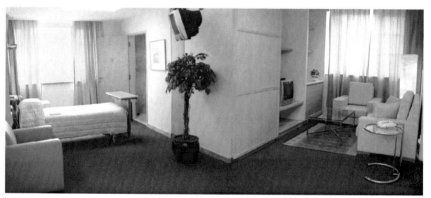

Raffles Hospital's five-star rooms and suites are available in a variety of sizes

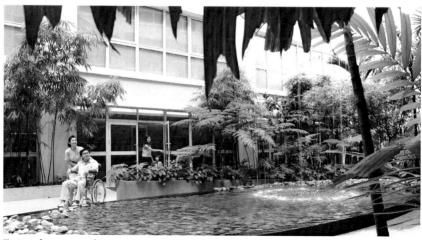

Enjoy the tranquil environment of Raffles Hospital Garden

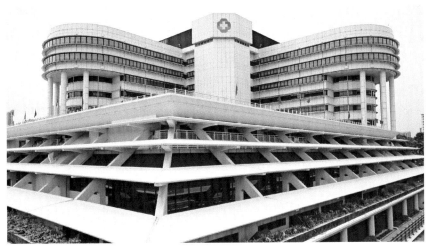

KK Women's and Children's Hospital

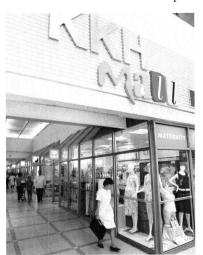

Shops at KK Hospital

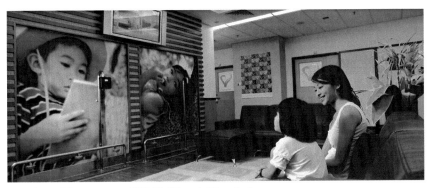

Family waiting room at KK Children's Hospital

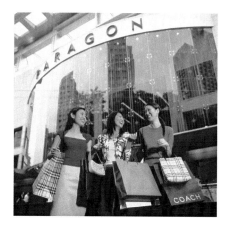

Orchard Road is the epicenter of Singapore's upscale shopping district, with swanky eateries and luxury hotels

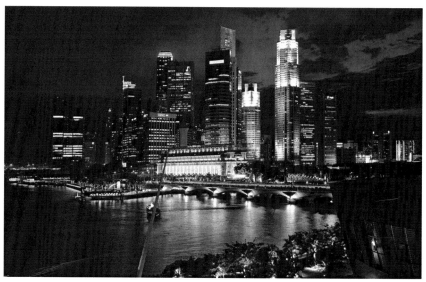

A view of Singapore's city lights — voted one of the world's best skylines

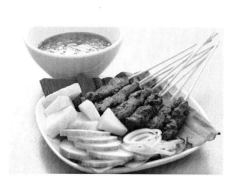

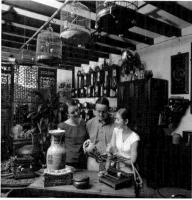

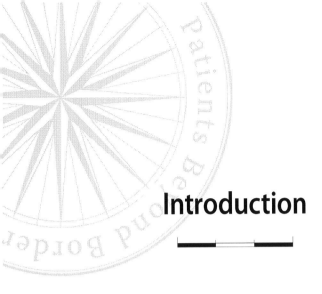

Introduction

Having read Part One, you now have a fair idea of what it takes to be a smart and informed health traveler. At this point, chances are you've already reached a decision about your course of treatment, and you may be seriously considering Singapore as a destination for your medical care.
Part Two, "Singapore: More Than a World-Class Health Destination," gives an overview of Singapore's initiatives, developments, and achievements as an international medical hub, and provides in-depth information about its leading healthcare establishments, health travel agents, and accommodations. It also includes a section of essential details for any Singapore-bound traveler.

Singapore: An Overview

History and Facts

Singapore is a former British Crown Colony and became an independent republic in 1965. Located at the tip of the Malay Peninsula in Southeast Asia, Singapore is made up of a main island with 63 surrounding islets, occupying a total land area of 272 square miles (704 square kilometers). With an airport served by more than 80 airlines with links to more than 180 cities in more than 50 countries, Singapore is one of the best-connected cities in the world.

Singapore has a total population of 4.5 million, consisting of 3.6 million residents and nearly a million expatriates from all over the globe. It is the second most densely populated country in the world after Monaco. Singapore's different ethnicities coexist in harmony; its population is 77 percent Chinese, 14 percent Malay, 8 percent Indian, and 1 percent other ethnicities.

Healthcare System

In 2000 the World Health Organization (WHO) ranked Singapore's healthcare system as the best in Asia and the sixth best in the world. Singapore provides the complete spectrum of healthcare services from primary care, such as health screening, to a broad range of specialist care services, such as organ transplantation, cardiothoracic surgery, and neurosurgery.

Singapore's life expectancy at birth is 79.3 years, 1.5 years longer than in the US. Its infant mortality rate of 1.9 per thousand and its near-zero maternal mortality rate are better than most countries in the world. These excellent healthcare indicators are achieved with a national healthcare expenditure that is less than 4 percent of the gross domestic product (GDP), of which the government contributes about one-third. In contrast, the US spends more than 16 percent of its GDP on healthcare.

There are 19 hospitals and national healthcare centers in Singapore. Of these, 13 are considered "public-sector" facilities. However, unique to most of the developed world, these public-sector hospitals are legally private limited companies and are licensed as private facilities under the Private Hospitals and Medical Clinics Act. Although wholly owned by the government, they are operated as private-sector entities to achieve the efficiency of the private sector in the public sector. These institutions are subsidized through a block grant from the government and held to a service level agreement. They are a far cry from what is commonly considered a "government hospital" in other countries.

Singapore has more than 6,500 doctors, 1,200 dentists, 19,000 nurses and midwives, and 1,200 pharmacists. Many doctors in Singapore trained internationally in the best centers in the world.

The accreditation par excellence for international healthcare facilities is issued by the Joint Commission International (JCI). At the time of this writing, most of Singapore's public- and private-sector institutions serving international patients are accredited by JCI — 13 in all. In 2006 JCI opened its Asia Pacific regional headquarters office in Singapore, enhancing Singapore's standing as a premier location for delivery of efficient, high-quality healthcare services.

The SingaporeMedicine Initiative —
Making Singapore a Regional Medical Hub

Launched in 2003, SingaporeMedicine is a multi-agency government initiative aimed at developing Singapore into a premier healthcare hub in Asia. Led by the Ministry of Health of Singapore, SingaporeMedicine is driven by three government agencies: the Economic Development Board (EDB), the Singapore Tourism Board (STB), and International Enterprise Singapore (IE Singapore).

EDB's role in SingaporeMedicine is to promote new investments and develop new capabilities in Singapore's healthcare industry. STB spearheads marketing, strengthens service delivery for international patients, and develops overseas referral channels. IE Singapore promotes the growth and expansion of Singapore's healthcare services in the region.

SingaporeMedicine builds upon the nation's well-established healthcare system and strong reputation for high-quality medicine. It also fits well with Singapore's growing biomedical sciences efforts in basic, translational, and clinical research. Critical to these efforts is the availability of a pool of skilled and experienced medical professionals and researchers, who are able to provide top-notch healthcare services and develop the next generation of cutting-edge treatments.

Medical Travel to Singapore

Why is it important to attract international patients to Singapore?

For its own citizens, Singapore has built its healthcare institutions and nationwide healthcare system to world-class standards. Paradoxically — and uniquely among countries receiving international medical travelers — Singapore serves international patients, in large part, to provide high-quality care to its local patients.

The Ministry of Health's comprehensive Health Manpower Development Programme sends doctors and other healthcare professionals to the best centers in the world for advanced training with high patient volumes in their subspecialties. Upon their return to Singapore, however, doctors often find that the small population of only 4.5 million offers few patients in their subspecialties. Similarly, hospitals also spend millions developing and acquiring the latest and best medical technologies, which are then underutilized by Singapore's small population.

To retain these extensively trained doctors — and continually develop and maintain their skills — and to support the ongoing acquisition and use of cutting-edge technologies, it is critical to have patient volumes commensurate with the medical services' level of sophistication. The addition of international patients allows Singapore's doctors to work in their subspecialties and enables hospitals' investments in advanced technologies to achieve cost-efficiency.

Why travel to Singapore for healthcare services?

✦ Regional Medical Hub

As a growing number of leading biomedical companies, including Eli Lilly, Novartis, MerLion, and ViaCell, have established regional headquarters in Singapore, the country is actively advancing the application of biomedical research in healthcare. World-class research capabilities in genomics, molecular biology, bioengineering, nanotechnology, and bioinformatics are already in place. Biopolis supports biomedical research and development activities, and Singapore has capabilities in basic and translational research, clinical trials, and healthcare delivery — from bench to bedside.

All of these activities enable Singapore's healthcare professionals to provide the latest innovative treatments and therapies, enhancing the country's reputation as a hub for healthcare in Asia.

✦ Hotspot for Medical Professionals

Because of its excellent pool of medical expertise and its first-rate healthcare infrastructure, Singapore attracts growing numbers of international medical professionals who come to learn, train, share, and network.

As the top convention city in Asia, Singapore plays host to significant numbers of international medical professionals who attend conferences, symposiums, and training seminars each year.

✦ International Patient Services

Because the healthcare facilities in Singapore have been receiving international patients for decades, services have been developed specifically for the international medical traveler. Healthcare providers assist their international patients with such services as visa renewals or travel arrangements for patients' companions. Patients and their families are met at the airport and well cared for until they board the plane to return home. Most healthcare facilities have an established International Patient Liaison Centre (IPLC) to cater to the special needs of medical travelers, even to the extent of arranging leisure activities, shopping, and dining.

✦ Peace of Mind

Ultimately, international patients are primarily concerned about their health and recovery. However, Singapore also meets all the other needs of medical travelers and their families. Singapore offers a comfortable and safe environment, low crime and high security, cultural and religious accommodation and acceptance, and convenient access and transportation.

The legal system in Singapore is reliable and well known for its impartiality and reliability. Political and Economic Risk Consultancy, Ltd. (PERC) rated Singapore's judicial system as the best in Asia, ahead of Hong Kong and Japan, in 2004; it also ranked Singapore at the top in consistency of application of laws. Singapore's legal system has also been praised by the International Monetary Fund and the Economist Intelligence Unit.

Singapore is a great tourist destination. It welcomed more than 10 million visitors in 2007 — more than two visitors for every citizen or permanent resident! Aside from healthcare, these visitors come to Singapore for shopping and leisure, business, and short- and long-term education. The companions of medical travelers are assured of having plenty to do and lots of fun.

A major worry for international patients is the cost of the trip — as well as possible additional costs arising from complications or unexpected events. Singapore's high-quality healthcare services ensure that patients are seen quickly and managed well, minimizing their hospital stay. Indeed, it is well known that although listed prices (such as cost per day) may be higher than at other destinations, the final bill in Singapore is often comparable or lower, because patients have better outcomes with lower complication rates and can be safely discharged within a shorter time without compromising safety. Singapore's Ministry of Health publishes average hospital costs on its Web site, www.moh.gov.sg.

In short, the medical traveler to Singapore will have little to worry about and can enjoy peace of mind when it matters most.

Singapore's Accreditation, Achievements, and Accolades

✦ Singapore has 13 JCI-accredited facilities.

✦ Singapore is recognized by WHO as having the safest blood

supply in the world, and it has been designated a WHO Collaborating Center for blood transfusion.

✦ 1983: Asia's first in vitro fertilization (IVF) baby was conceived in Singapore.

✦ 1985: Asia's first gamete intrafallopian transfer (GIFT) baby was conceived in Singapore.

✦ 1987: Singapore produced the world's first frozen-embryo baby.

✦ 1988: The world's first micromanipulation baby (SUZI) was conceived in Singapore.

✦ 1991: The world's first human tubal coculture baby was conceived in Singapore.

✦ 1992: The world's first blastocyst transfer baby was conceived in Singapore.

✦ 1995: Singapore physicians performed the world's first successful peripheral blood stem cell transplant from an unrelated donor on a patient with thalassemia major.

✦ 2000: WHO ranked Singapore's healthcare system as the best in Asia and the sixth best in the world.

✦ 2001: Singapore surgeons separated a pair of craniopagus (joined at the head) conjoined twins from Nepal.

✦ 2001: Singapore physicians performed the world's first successful cord blood transplant from an unrelated donor on a patient with thalassemia major.

✦ 2001: Singapore physicians performed Southeast Asia's first heart transplant using a left ventricular assist device (LVAD), an electronic device that gives critically ill heart patients new hope while waiting for a suitable heart.

✦ 2002: Singapore physicians performed Southeast Asia's first unrelated adult living donor liver transplant.

✦ 2003: Singapore was the first country in the region to acquire a positron emission tomography/computed tomography (PET/CT) scanner.

✦ 2004: Singapore physicians and dentists performed a revolutionary two-stage "tooth-in-eye" surgical procedure, Southeast Asia's first, restoring a blind boy's sight.

✦ 2005: Singapore physicians performed Asia's first "kidney cum bone marrow" transplant.

✦ 2005: Singapore physicians achieved a breakthrough with stem cells in a clinical trial to treat defects in knee cartilage.

✦ 2005: Singapore physicians performed Asia's first Delta Reversed Shoulder Replacement, a technique to relieve pain and return function to patients with shoulder arthritis due to rotator cuff tears.

✦ 2007: Singapore implemented the world's first BrainSUITE, a digitally integrated neuroscience center with an operating theater equipped to perform MRI and CT during surgery.

The Medical Traveler's Essentials

Airport Tax

A passenger service charge of SGD21 (Singapore dollars; see below) is typically incorporated in your airfare ticket. If this has not been done, you are required to pay the SGD21 upon check-in at the airport. In certain instances, some airlines may absorb this service charge.

Banking

Banking hours are Monday through Friday, from 1000 hrs to 1500 hrs; and Saturday, from 0930 hrs to 1300 hrs (some banks are open until 1500 hrs).

Most banks offer, and cash, traveler's checks and change foreign currencies. Passports are required when cashing traveler's checks. A nominal commission may be charged.

Country Code

The country code for Singapore is 65. There is no area code. To make an international call to Singapore, dial the international access code followed by 65 and the Singapore telephone number.

Credit/Charge Cards

Major credit cards are widely accepted by establishments in Singapore.

American Express:	65 6880.1111
Diners Club:	65 6416.0800
JCB:	65 6734.0206
MasterCard:	65 800 110.0113 (toll-free)
Visa:	65 800 448.1250 (toll-free)

Currency

The national currency is Singapore dollars (SGD) and cents. All merchants and service providers accept Singapore dollars. Euros, US and Australian dollars, yen, and British pounds are also accepted in most major shopping centers and department stores.

Drinking Water

It is perfectly safe to drink water straight from the tap in Singapore. However, for those medical travelers who prefer bottled water, local supermarkets and grocers usually carry a sizeable range.

Drug Policies

Illegal drug use and illicit trafficking in narcotics and psychotropic substances is strictly prohibited in Singapore and will be dealt with seriously.

Electricity

Singapore's voltage is 220–240 volts AC, 50 cycles per second. On request, most hotels will provide transformers to visitors with electrical appliances of a different voltage. The power plugs used in Singapore are of the three-pin, square-shaped type.

Mobile Phones

The two mobile phone networks are GSM900 and GSM1800; the three mobile phone service providers are SingTel, M1, and StarHub. For making international calls, the access codes are 001, 013, or 019 for SingTel, 002 or 021 for M1, and 008 or 018 for StarHub.

Money Changers

Money can be changed at banks and hotels and wherever the sign "Licensed Money Changer" is displayed. Most shopping centers have licensed money changers.

Pay Phone Services

Public pay phones can be found in most shopping complexes and train stations. Local calls are charged at 10 Singapore cents per three minutes. Stored-value phone-cards in denominations of SGD2, SGD5, SGD10, SGD20, and SGD50 can be purchased from post offices and phone-card agents. To make an international call, dial the access code followed by the country code, area code, and telephone number. International calling cards in denominations of SGD10, SGD20, and SGD50 are also available at Singapore Changi Airport, 7-Eleven stores, all post offices, and other retail outlets.

Postal Services

Singapore Post operates an extensive network of postal outlets conveniently located throughout the country. Most postal outlets are open Monday through Friday from 0830 hrs to 1700 hrs, and until 1300 hrs on Saturday.

Smoking

Smoking is not permitted in public service vehicles, museums, libraries, elevators, theaters, cinemas, air-conditioned restaurants, hair salons, supermarkets, department stores, or government offices. In accordance with efforts to improve the nightlife experience for all, smoking is no longer allowed in pubs, discos, or other night spots, except within designated smoking rooms or smoking corners.

Tipping

Tipping is not practiced, because most hotels and restaurants in Singapore already levy a 10 percent service charge on customers' bills. Cabs are metered, and there is no need to add a tip beyond the meter reading. However, certain surcharges may apply, depending on when and where the taxi is taken. These may vary by cab company and are usually detailed on a sign within the vehicle.

Visa and Entry

Generally, foreigners who do not require visas for entry and are visiting as tourists will be given social visit passes for up to 30 days upon their arrival in Singapore.

What to Wear

Singapore's climate is warm and humid throughout the year, with a daily average temperature range of 75–90 degrees Fahrenheit (24–32 degrees Celsius). Light, summer clothing of natural fabrics (such as cotton) is best for everyday wear. Casual dress is acceptable for most situations and occasions, but some establishments may require something more formal. It is always advisable to check beforehand about dress regulations.

Useful Telephone Numbers

Police	999 (toll-free)
Emergencies/Ambulance/Fire Brigade	995 (toll-free)
Citysearch (operator-assisted Yellow Pages)	1 900 777.7777
Changi Airport Flight Information	1 800 542.4422
Taxi Services:	
Centralized Dial-A-Cab System	6 DIAL.CAB
Comfort Citycab	6552.1111
Comfort Premier Cab	6552.2828
Premier Taxis	6363.6888
SMRT Taxis	6555.8888
Smart Automobile	6485.7777
International Calls (operator-assisted)	104
Time of Day	1711
Weather Information	6542.7788
Singapore Tourism Board Touristline (24-hour automated tourist information system)	1 800 736.2000 (toll-free)

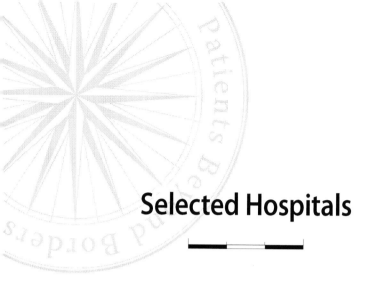

Selected Hospitals

AsiaMedic Specialist Centre

350 Orchard Road
#08-00 Shaw House
SINGAPORE 238868
Tel: 65 6789.8888
Fax: 65 6738.4136
Email: info@asiamedic.com.sg
Web: www.asiamedic.com.sg

Listed and ranked in 2007's *Singapore 1000* published by DP Information Group, AsiaMedic Specialist Centre (AsiaMedic) is a premier, one-stop healthcare and preventive medicine service provider. Focusing on prevention and early illness detection, AsiaMedic utilizes cutting-edge medical technology in specialized clinical services. Its strength lies in offering niche and advanced healthcare services in a non-hospital environment.

AsiaMedic's specialty centers offer personalized health screening, medical aesthetics, and diagnostic services in a comfortable outpatient setting. These centers are managed by teams of highly trained and dedicated physicians, radiologists, technologists, and administrative personnel. As a strong advocate of preventive care, AsiaMedic gears its services toward accurate diagnosis with efficient and effective use of time.

AsiaMedic's centers of excellence include

✦ **PET/CT Centre,** among the first in Singapore to introduce an integrated positron emission tomography (PET) and computerized tomography (CT) scanner for highly accurate detection and localization of early-stage cancer tumors. Launched in 2003, the center focuses on oncology (lung, breast, testicular, ovarian, and colorectal cancers, lymphomas, melanomas, and recurrent brain tumors); cardiology (coronary artery disease and myocardial viability); neurology (Parkinson's, Alzheimer's, Huntington's, epilepsy, multiple sclerosis, and stroke); and psychiatry.

✦ **Advanced Imaging Services,** providing a wide range of diagnostic radiological examinations, including general radiology, CT scanning, magnetic resonance imaging (MRI), mammography, ultrasound, bone densitometry, fluoroscopy, and intravenous urography — all conveniently centralized on the same premises. This center boasts Singapore's first Signa Infinity 1.5T MRI scanner, offering ultra-fast and ultra-sharp diagnostic imaging capability.

✦ **AsiaMedic Eye Centre,** a regional leader in eye care and vision correction. Most surgeries are performed under local anesthesia and usually do not require a hospital stay. The center also offers special screening examinations to detect various eye diseases. One of the first non-hospital eye centers to introduce a twin-laser correction system for presbyopia (refraction problems in older adults), it also introduced Singapore's first EpiLASIK (to cut very thin corneal flaps) and keratoplasty (near vision correction without corneal cuts).

✢ **Aesthetic Medical Centre,** offering plastic and cosmetic surgery and other procedures for the face and body. Skin treatments include laser with intense pulsed light technology, Botox, chemical peels, and collagen injections. Body-contouring techniques include Endermologie for cellulite removal, liposuction, breast augmentation, breast lift, and breast reduction.

✢ **Wellness Assessment Centre,** a one-stop screening center focusing on holistic well-being and combining all of the required laboratory and radiology tests under one roof. Comprehensive health screening programs are customized to identify patients' risk factors by their gender and age group; thereafter, health-maintenance and treatment plans can be tailored to achieve optimal health.

Mount Alvernia Hospital

International Patients Service Assistance
820 Thomson Road
SINGAPORE 574623
Tel: 65 6347.6666
Fax: 65 6255.6303
Email: intpt@mtalvernia-hospital.org
Web: www.mtalvernia-hospital.org

Mount Alvernia Hospital (MAH) is a private, acute-care hospital that has built a reputation over the last 45 years for high-quality, affordable, and personalized healthcare services. It attained ISO 9001:2000 certification in 1996. MAH offers a comprehensive range of medical specialties, and the hospital's four specialized centers consolidate resources and expertise in key medical fields to address patients' individual needs.

MAH's centers of excellence include

✦ **Brain Centre,** with an experienced team of specialists, therapists, and nurses who take a multidisciplinary approach to the diagnosis, treatment, and rehabilitation of patients with neurological disorders. In addition to diagnostic testing, the center offers medical, surgical, post-operative, and rehabilitative care for a wide range of conditions, including brain and spinal tumors, stroke, blood vessel disorders and aneurysms, hydrocephalus, neck pain and cervical spondylosis, spinal disc ailments, epilepsy, Alzheimer's and Parkinson's diseases, and others.

✦ **Heart Centre,** where experienced cardiothoracic surgeons and cardiologists provide a full range of services from preventive care to surgery. The cardiovascular laboratory boasts one of the latest angiography machines, with advanced capabilities facilitating coronary and vascular tests. The center also performs invasive diagnostic and therapeutic procedures, including treatment for acute myocardial infarction, in addition to intra-aortic balloon counterpulsation for patients with low blood pressure. Open-heart surgeries include coronary artery bypass graft, heart valve repair and replacement, open thoracic aortic surgery, endovascular aortic stenting, congenital heart surgery, and endoscopic harvesting of the saphenous vein and radial artery.

✦**Minimally Invasive Surgery Centre,** practicing and researching less-invasive surgical techniques that offer quicker recovery and fewer long-term consequences. Minimal access techniques rely on a camera-equipped telescope or endoscope placed through a small incision, allowing the surgeon to view the surgical site on a monitor and operate by manipulating small instruments through two to four other small incisions. The specialists at MAH use these techniques in most fields of surgery.

✦**Sports Medicine and Sports Surgery Centre,** providing cost-effective management of musculoskeletal injuries. Through comprehensive sports medicine services that include medical consultation, rehabilitation, injury prevention, surgery, exercise management, nutrition, and education, the center's personnel help patients of all ages achieve a lifetime of participation in sports, exercise, and physical activity. Facilities include private consultation rooms, electrotherapy treatment, massage cubicles, extracorporeal shock wave therapy (ESWT), and a modern exercise gymnasium with state-of-the-art cardiovascular and strength training equipment. The center's diagnostic imaging department is equipped with MRI, CT, x-ray, and ultrasound systems.

Specialties

✦ Cardiology, cardiothoracic surgery, dental/oral maxillofacial surgery, otolaryngology, endocrinology, gastroenterology, geriatric medicine, hematology, neurology and neurosurgery, obstetrics and gynecology, oncology, ophthalmology, orthopedic surgery, pediatric medicine and neonatology, pediatric surgery, plastic and reconstructive surgery, renal medicine, rheumatology, and urology

Services Provided for International Patients

✦ Appointment and referral scheduling and confirmation

✦ Travel planning

✦ Accommodations arrangement

✦ Airport pickup and transportation

✦ Arrangements for direct admission

✦ Assistance before, during, and after hospitalization

✦ Assistance with billing inquiries

✦ Assistance with sightseeing and tourism inquiries

✦ Evacuation and repatriation assistance

Feature Story

Neurosurgery for a Brain Aneurysm Saves the Life of a Vietnamese Woman

In February 2006, 27-year-old Vietnamese architect Ms. Doan Thi Thu Hong suddenly developed severe headaches followed by vomiting. She was admitted to a hospital in Hanoi and diagnosed with a brain hemorrhage. The source was an aneurysm, a weak spot in an artery, seated deep in the brain and difficult to reach. Doctors attempted non-operative treatment, such as inserting a stent and coils into the affected area, but without success.

Ms. Doan then had more episodes of bleeding, with the third so severe that she was put on a ventilator. Her doctors said there was nothing more they could do and advised her husband to take her home. Refusing to give up, he contacted a neurosurgeon in Ho Chi Minh City, who referred the couple to Dr. Timothy Lee at Mount Alvernia Hospital. In June Ms. Doan arrived in Singapore, where doctors at Mount Alvernia attempted another non-operative treatment, but to no avail. Surgery was the only option.

Dr. Lee enlisted the help of an ear, nose, and throat surgeon to access Ms. Doan's brain from behind the ear; he also employed the standard approach of entering the front of the brain. The doctors first inserted a small tube to divert accumulated fluid, carefully divided a major vein to get closer to the aneurysm, and then clipped the artery. An angiogram confirmed the procedure was a success.

Ms. Doan recovered well from the surgery and had no neurological problems other than initial giddiness, which gradually subsided. After three months, she was completely well and returned home. Her husband says, "We are extremely grateful to the doctor who performed this 'impossible' operation. Through the media, we want to provide information about our case so that others in the same situation can keep their hopes alive. We were very impressed with the skills and level of care provided by Dr. Lee and Mount Alvernia Hospital. We would not have been able to survive if we had not sought treatment in Singapore."

NATIONAL HEALTHCARE GROUP

6 Commonwealth Lane
Level 6, GMTI Building
SINGAPORE 149437
Tel: 65 6779.2777 (24-hour hotline)
Fax: 65 6777.8065
Email: iplc@nhg.com.sg
Web: www.nhg.com.sg

National Healthcare Group (NHG) is a major public healthcare provider in Singapore, recognized at home and abroad for its medical expertise and high-quality facilities. Singapore's first healthcare group to have one of its centers achieve JCI accreditation, NHG currently includes several JCI-accredited hospitals and centers.

NHG's institutions provide a full range of healthcare from health screening to tertiary specialist services. A one-stop **International Patient Liaison Centre (IPLC)** facilitates health travelers' access to all of the group's services. The IPLC also acts as a liaison between NHG and referral resources, patients and families, and payers outside of Singapore.

As a major healthcare provider in Singapore, NHG offers an integrated network of nine primary polyclinics, three acute-care hospitals, one psychiatric hospital, one national center, three specialty institutes, and five business divisions.

Member institutions include **Alexandra Hospital*, National University Hospital*, Tan Tock Seng Hospital*, Institute of Mental Health/Woodbridge Hospital*, Johns Hopkins Singapore International Medical Centre*, National Skin Centre*, The Cancer Institute, The Eye Institute,** and **The Heart Institute.** (* JCI-accredited.)

Services Provided for International Patients

✦ Appointment scheduling

✦ Flight reservations and confirmations

✦ Accommodations arrangement

✦ Airport pickup and transportation

✦ Arrangements for direct admission

✦ Assistance before, during, and after hospitalization

✦ Medical referrals

✦ Language translation

✦ Liaison with employers and insurance companies

✦ Sightseeing arrangements (such as restaurant reservations and ticket purchases)

✦ Assistance with visa extensions

✦ Evacuation and repatriation assistance

Feature Story

From the Tundra to the Tropics for Treatment

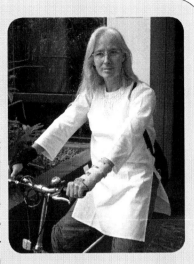

An avid mountaineer, 50-year-old Sangeet Kaur Khalsa had constant pain in her knee. A surgeon she saw in California suspected a meniscal tear, but she postponed further investigation after learning that the required MRI scan would cost her US$2,500. "I was just not prepared to pay so much for that," Khalsa recalls. "Back home in Alaska, it was even higher, around US$3,700. I sank into despair, not knowing where I could get good treatment and afford it."

Searching for options abroad, she came across the Web site of Overseas Medical Services, Canada, Inc. (see the "Health Travel Agents" section) and spoke with Ms. Aruna Th-Hollingshead, who assisted her all the way through the process. She admits, "I was a little skeptical at first, but then Aruna called and said she had found a doctor for me at Singapore's National University Hospital."

In addition to making Khalsa's travel arrangements, Aruna provided information about the hospital and the doctor who would treat her. There was, however, a little problem. Most countries will not issue a visa to travelers whose passports have less than six months left before expiry — and Khalsa's passport was expiring in four.

Aruna relates, "The people at NUH sorted out her visa with the immigration department in no time. They clearly took pains to make things easier. This is important for patients like Khalsa, because they have to endure their physical pain on top of the disappointment of their health-care system. They don't need further headaches."

In May 2007, Khalsa arrived at Changi International Airport, breezed through immigration, and was brought by NUH staff to the hospital, where she found welcoming orchids in her room. Dr. James Hui Hoi Po, associate professor and senior consultant in the Department of Orthopaedic Surgery, met with Khalsa to outline the diagnostic and treatment plan.

The next day, the long-awaited MRI scan (which only cost about US$500) confirmed that a meniscal tear was the source of the pain. To solve the problem, Dr. Hui trimmed Khalsa's meniscus and smoothed the inside of the kneecap. The 45-minute procedure proceeded without any complications.

Within a few days after her surgery, Khalsa was a common sight scooting around the hospital and was looking forward to scaling the mountains back home again. She reports, "Dr. Hui and the other doctors took pains to explain things and kept me informed of every-thing. The nurses spoilt me. The healthcare system as a whole is really remarkable."

Alexandra Hospital

International Patient Services
378 Alexandra Road
Level 3, Administration Block
SINGAPORE 159964
Tel: 65 6476.8828
Fax: 65 6379.5348
Email: ips@alexhosp.com.sg
Web: www.alexhosp.com.sg

Formerly the British Military Hospital, Alexandra Hospital received a complete makeover in 2000 under the auspices of NHG. Besides offering patient-centered service and promoting medical excellence through its research infrastructure, the hospital prides itself on its tranquil and healing environment. Because research shows that greenery speeds recovery, the hospital offers patients a therapeutic garden that includes a 100-species butterfly trail, an ecological garden, a fragrant garden, and even a medicinal garden with 100 types of healing plants.

Alexandra Hospital also believes in driving innovation and quality through learning from other industries, such as hospitality, manufacturing, and telecommunications. One innovation at Alexandra Hospital is a platform that allows post-surgery patients to update nurses about their condition by sending pictures of their wounds via multimedia message service or email.

Specialties

✦ Cardiology, dentistry, diabetes (diagnosis and treatment), endocrinology, gastroenterology, general surgery, neurology, ophthalmology, orthopedics, and neck and head surgery

Achievements

✦ JCI accreditation in 2005

✦ ISO 9001:2000 (Quality Management System) and ISO 14001: 1996 (Environmental Management System) certifications

✦ College of American Pathologists accreditation

✦ ISO Occupational Health and Safety Management Systems Award

✦ Asian Hospital Management Award of "Most Outstanding in Customer Service" in 2006

✦ Southeast Asia's first limb reattachment

National University Hospital

International Patient Liaison Centre
5 Lower Kent Ridge Road
Level 3, Kent Ridge Wing
SINGAPORE 119074
Tel: 65 6779.2777 (24-hour helpline)
Fax: 65 6777.8065
Email: iplc@nhg.com.sg
Web: www.nuh.com.sg

National University Hospital (NUH) is an acute-care tertiary hospital. NUH offers a full range of services and facilities, including specialist clinics and centers, clinical support services (such as dietetics and diagnostic imaging), dental services (including oral and maxillofacial surgery), nursing care, and support groups (such as the Liver Transplant Support Group, Breast Cancer Support Group, and Children's Cancer Foundation).

Being a university hospital allows NUH to translate the latest clinical research into advanced treatments. Its many clinicians also serve on the National University of Singapore's Faculty of Medicine. These dual roles enable them to stay abreast of developments in skills and technology, as well as to participate in research on new cures and treatments.

NUH ensures high standards through constant monitoring and tracking clinical quality indicators across departments. This has resulted in excellent clinical outcomes, such as an improved cure rate for acute lymphocytic leukemia from 62 percent in 1988–1996 to 84 percent in 1997–2002; a significantly better three-year overall survival rate (74 percent versus 35 percent) and disease-free survival rate (83 percent versus 31 percent) for acute myelogenous leukemia; an improved survival rate for stomach cancer (69 percent versus 60 percent); and a 100 percent success rate for extracapsular cataract extraction.

In early 2008, the Hannaford Bros. supermarket chain made a special arrangement with NHG. Any Hannaford Bros. employee can get a hip replacement done at Singapore's National University Hospital, and Hannaford Bros. will cover the entire US$8,000 tab — including travel expenses for the patient and spouse.

Specialties

✦ Cardiology, cardiothoracic and vascular surgery, gastroenterology and hepatology, hematology, oncology, hand and reconstructive microsurgery, neonatology, obstetrics and gynecology, ophthalmology, orthopedic surgery, head and neck surgery, pathology, pediatric surgery, urology, oral and maxillofacial surgery, and restorative dentistry

Achievements

✦ First hospital in Singapore to obtain JCI accreditation, August 2004

✦ Singapore's first and only simultaneous triple ISO certification: ISO 9001:2000 (Quality Management System), ISO 14001:1996 (Environmental Management System), and OHSAS 18001:1999 (Occupational Health and Safety Management System)

✦ Asia's first frozen-embryo baby

✦ World's first cord blood transplant from an unrelated donor for thalassemia major

✦ American Society of Hematology Merit Award to NUH researcher and pediatrician in biomedical research on childhood acute lymphoblastic leukemia

✦ Breakthrough in stem cell clinical trial to treat defects in knee cartilage

✦ Asia's first Delta Reversed Shoulder System (technique to relieve pain and return function to patients who have shoulder arthritis due to rotator cuff tears)

✦ Asia's first middle ear implant

✦ Asia's first hip resurfacing procedure

Feature Story

Singapore Was the Right Choice for Me

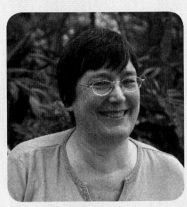

In early December 2007, 53-year-old Londoner Jane B. experienced a nagging pain in her lower abdomen and suspected something was wrong. A pelvic ultrasound and a CT scan revealed ovarian cysts and also an unidentified mass within the cysts. When Jane underwent surgery to remove both ovaries, the pathology results indicated a benign tumor in the left ovary and signs of a borderline tumor malignancy in the right.

"I was shocked when I learnt I had ovarian cancer," she recalls. Another operation was necessary, a bigger one, with a longer recovery period. "When my doctors suggested I head to Singapore, I was comforted, as I was aware of its reputation for good medical service. I had no reservations about it."

Her London doctors contacted Singapore's National University Hospital and put her in touch with Dr. Jeffery Low, head of the Department of Gynecologic Oncology and Urogynecology and a senior consultant in obstetrics and gynecology. Jane corresponded with Dr. Low via email, and he detailed the operation she was to undergo. She also contacted NUH's International Patient Liaison Centre, where the staff took care of administrative details for her trip and arranged with a nursing home for her post-surgery recuperation.

Jane arrived in Singapore in February 2008. After a complete physical examination, chest x-ray, mammogram, and blood tests, the plan was to remove her uterus, take a fluid sample from her abdomen, and biopsy any areas where the cancer might have spread. Dr. Low says, "This was to help determine the precise stage of her cancer, so we could provide her with an accurate prognosis and decide if there was a need for chemotherapy."

The two-hour surgery showed that her cancer was, fortunately, at an early stage. The next day, Jane's nurses coaxed her out of bed to do some simple exercises. By the fourth day post-surgery, she was on her feet and walking short distances unassisted. A few days later, she was transferred to Econ Medicare Centre, where she continued her rehabilitation for four weeks.

Jane relates, "In Singapore, everyone speaks English, which was a relief. The level of service and care at NUH was excellent. Even at the nursing home, I was made to feel very comfortable and, besides daily physiotherapy, I had acupuncture to help me relax. It was great." Eager to get back to her work and social life, Jane was finally given a clean bill of health in March 2008.

Tan Tock Seng Hospital

International Patient Liaison Centre
11 Jalan Tan Tock Seng, Level 1
SINGAPORE 308433
Tel: 65 6779.2777 (24-hour helpline)
Fax: 65 6777.8065
Email: iplc@nhg.com.sg
Web: www.ttsh.com.sg

Established in 1844, Tan Tock Seng Hospital (TTSH) is Singapore's second largest acute-care hospital, with 1,400 beds. With strengths in geriatric medicine, infectious disease management, rehabilitation medicine, respiratory medicine, rheumatology, allergy, and immunology, TTSH is also a major referral center for diagnostic radiology, emergency medicine, ophthalmology, gastroenterology, otolaryngology, and orthopedic surgery.

The hospital includes two major specialty centers: one in rehabilitation medicine and communicable diseases, and the other in research on treatments for emerging diseases.

The hospital's **Ophthalmology Department,** the second largest in Singapore, is under the NHG umbrella of The Eye Institute (TEI@TTSH; see below). TEI@TTSH offers the full range of tertiary ophthalmic care at one location and utilizes cutting-edge technologies for optimal outcomes. It was the first in Asia to use IntraLase technology in LASIK surgery without a mechanical blade; to perform macular translocation surgery; to offer 23-gauge vitrectomy surgery; and to offer implantable contact lenses as an alternative for patients unsuitable for LASIK.

Specialties

✦ Cardiology, clinical epidemiology, diagnostic radiology, endocrinology, gastroenterology, geriatric medicine, infectious diseases, ophthalmology, orthopedic surgery, otolaryngology, rheumatology, allergy and immunology, and urology

Achievements

✦ JCI accreditation in August 2005

✦ ISO 9001:2000 (Quality Management System) and ISO 14001: 1996 (Environmental Management System) certifications

✦ Singapore's first hospital to offer stereotactic MRI-guided thalamotomy for Parkinson's disease

✦ Asia's first Fitbone surgery

Institute of Mental Health/ Woodbridge Hospital

10 Buangkok View
Buangkok Green Medical Park
SINGAPORE 539747
Tel: 65 6389.2222 (24-hour helpline)
Fax: 65 6385.1050
Email: enquiry@imh.com.sg
Web: www.imh.com.sg

The Institute of Mental Health (IMH) is a 2,369-bed, acute- and chronic-care, tertiary psychiatric hospital that offers a multi-faceted and comprehensive range of psychiatric services for children and adolescents, adults, and the elderly. The hospital's nursing, clinical psychology, occupational therapy, and medical social work departments support a multidisciplinary approach to patient care. Its specially designed landscape provides psychiatric patients with a serene, non-hospital environment to aid in their healing. IMH obtained JCI accreditation in 2005.

Specialties

✦ General psychiatry, child and adolescent psychiatry, community psychiatry, geriatric psychiatry, forensic psychiatry, early psychosis intervention, addiction medicine, mood disorders, sleep disorders, and sexual dysfunction

Johns Hopkins Singapore International Medical Centre

11 Jalan Tan Tock Seng
SINGAPORE 308433
Tel: 65 6880.2236
Fax: 65 6880.2223
Email: iploffice@imc.jhmi.edu
Web: www.imc.jhmi.edu

Johns Hopkins Singapore International Medical Centre (JHS) was established in 1998 by the American university of the same name as its base of medical operations in Southeast Asia. The center concentrates on patient care, education, and research. In 2004 JHS became the first healthcare facility in Singapore to receive JCI accreditation.

JHS provides Hopkins-quality oncology services to local and international patients. JHS uses the most up-to-date therapies and new technologies, working in collaboration with researchers at Johns Hopkins University, Johns Hopkins School of Medicine, National University of Singapore, and National University Hospital. JHS physicians collaborate with Singapore medical institutions and physicians to provide inpatient management and treatment of disease; outpatient care to screen for, diagnose, monitor, and treat early and advanced cancers; second opinions on complex medical conditions; and consultations with referring physicians.

Research and educational activities are carried out by the **Division of Biomedical Sciences,** an academic division of the medical school, with a focus on cellular and immunotherapy and a specific interest in stem cell, virology, and cancer research.

Specialties

✦ All types of cancer, including breast, ovarian, uterine, cervical, lung, throat, nasopharynx, stomach, liver, colon, lymphoma, myeloma, prostate, bladder, and kidney

National Skin Centre

1 Mandalay Road
SINGAPORE 308205
Tel: 65 6235.4455
Fax: 65 6253.3225
Email: appointment@nsc.gov.sg
Web: www.nsc.gov.sg

Accredited by JCI in 2007, The National Skin Centre provides specialized dermatological services and conducts research in dermatology. In addition to being the national and regional referral center for treatment of complex skin diseases, it is a training center for local and international skin specialists and paramedical personnel. The center offers clinics for contact dermatitis, joint occupational dermatoses, cutaneous infection, dermatological and laser surgery, drug eruption, hair and nail, immunodermatology, lymphoma, pediatric dermatology, phototherapy, and wounds and ulcers.

The Cancer Institute

TCI@Alexandra Hospital
TCI@National University Hospital
TCI@Tan Tock Seng Hospital
Tel: 65 6779.2777 (24-hour hotline)
Email: iplc@nhg.com.sg
Web: www.tci.nhg.com.sg

The Cancer Institute (TCI) was established to provide comprehensive cancer management from prevention to recovery and long-term health maintenance. TCI links various medical facilities and streamlines their integrated care process. The institute's aim is to reduce cancer mortality and enhance quality of life by preventing cancer and providing treatment and care through progressive efforts in service, education, and research.

The Eye Institute

TEI@Alexandra Hospital
TEI@National University Hospital
TEI@Tan Tock Seng Hospital
TTSH LASIK Centre
Tel: 65 6779.2777 (24-hour hotline)
Email: iplc@nhg.com.sg
Web: www.tei.nhg.com.sg

The Eye Institute (TEI) was established to meet the increasing demand for eye services. It integrates opthalmological clinical expertise and facilities across NHG institutions. Ten subspecialties within TEI's services address all aspects of eye disease and treatment. TEI treats cataracts with modern methods that produce high success rates.

The Heart Institute

Department of Cardiac, Thoracic, and Vascular Surgery
5 Lower Kent Ridge Road
Level 2, Main Building
SINGAPORE 119074
Tel: 65 6779.2777 (24-hour hotline)
Fax: 65 6778.6057
Email: iplc@nhg.com.sg
Web: www.thi.nhg.com.sg

The Heart Institute (THI) combines the resources and expertise of several NHG institutions in cardiology, cardiothoracic surgery, and vascular surgery to provide a seamless continuum of care for heart patients. The various cardiac units work closely with the polyclinics and general practitioners to provide cost-efficient clinical care from inpatient treatment to outpatient cardiac support, including rehabilitation and primary cardiac care.

Pacific Healthcare

290 Orchard Road
#19-01 Paragon
SINGAPORE 238859
Tel: 65 6887.3737 (24-hour hotline)
Fax: 65 6887.1292
Email: customerservice@pachealthholdings.com
Web: www.pachealthholdings.com

Pacific Healthcare (PacHealth) is an integrated healthcare provider offering a comprehensive range of services encompassing specialist medical care, general practice medicine, dentistry, health screening, and wellness services. With a team of more than 100 dedicated medical professionals and a wide network of clinics and facilities, PacHealth focuses on the holistic health and well-being of patients and takes a multidisciplinary approach to treatment. Its core competencies include cosmetic surgery and aesthetic medicine, obstetrics and gynecology, and dental implantation and aesthetic dentistry.

PacHealth operates two nursing homes, a day-surgery center, and a psychiatric hospital. Its centers of excellence include

+ **Specialist Surgical and Laser Centre,** a day-surgery center with five operating theaters equipped with HEPA air-filtration ventilation systems to ensure a surgically clean environment. The center also has six recovery bays equipped with oxygen panels and monitoring equipment.

+ **Pacific Healthcare Specialist Centre,** providing a diverse multidisciplinary range of medical and dental specialties, such as anti-aging treatments, dermatology, plastic surgery and aesthetics, dentistry (general, cosmetic, and implant), pediatrics, health screening, obstetrics and gynecology, respiratory and internal medicine, and reconstructive microsurgery of the hand and wrist.

+ **Wellness Lounge,** an aesthetics and wellness center that complements PacHealth's integrated specialist center and day-surgery center. The lounge provides a comprehensive range of facial and body-contouring treatments for men and women. Professional consultants customize skin and body treatments for each patient.

✦ **Medical and Dental Centre,** providing general dental treatment, endodontics, orthodontics, periodontics, prosthodontics, occlusal rehabilitation, pedodontics, oral surgery, dental implants, aesthetic dentistry, and dental appliances and prostheses. The center also has a medical clinic providing health screening programs, medical consultations, and cosmetic medicine.

Feature Story

I Found My Lost Years in Singapore

Even for those blessed with "good genes," age lines appear and the face loses its youthful glow. Some people are resigned to this; others, like 49-year old Catherine Mae of Melbourne, Australia, begin to rue their fading youth. "I was at the stage of my life when I felt that my face could do with a little freshening up. I was trying to figure out exactly what I would need, but to be honest, I didn't know," she admits.

In talking with friends and reading up on available treatments, she noticed that one name often cropped up: one of Singapore's leading dermatologists, the US-trained Dr. Patricia Yuen, consultant dermatologist at Singapore's Pacific Healthcare Specialist Centre. Catherine headed for Singapore and met with Dr. Yuen. She relates, "I hadn't expected it, but Dr. Yuen was naturally warm and friendly, and oozed confidence, which was totally reassuring. When I asked her what I needed done, she just looked at me intently and then cited a list of things that would help me achieve the look I was hoping for."

For the next three hours, Catherine underwent a series of treatments. Dr. Yuen outlines, "For her wrinkles and fine lines, I used Botox to relax the muscles and diminish the lines. Since she wanted her tired skin to look refreshed and rejuvenated, we also did microdermabrasion and vitamin C iontophoresis combined with laser to help brighten her complexion and address her problem of rosacea, which are the visible red capillaries on her face." Iontophoresis involves applying a vitamin C serum followed by a very low-level electrical current to increase the vitamin's depth of penetration.

Dr. Yuen's clientele includes professionals, celebrities, and even heads-of-state; she estimates that up to 20 percent of her patients fly to Singapore specially to see her for various skin conditions and aesthetic treatments.

Catherine found that with her rejuvenated look, the compliments started to flow. She says, "This whole makeover has definitely had a positive effect on all aspects of my life. Although I'm not too thrilled about turning 50, I'm certainly happier with how I look and feel now: fresh, recharged, and youthful. It's like I found my lost years in Singapore."

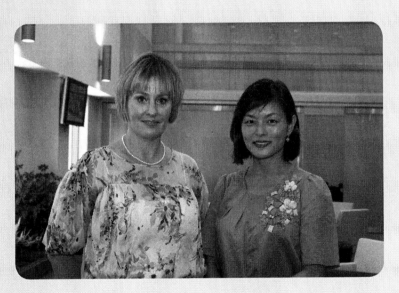

PARKWAY GROUP HEALTHCARE

International Patient Assistance Centre
83 Clemenceau Avenue
#10-05/06/07 UE Square
SINGAPORE 239920
Tel: 65 6735.5000 (24-hour hotline)
Fax: 65 6732.6733
Email: ipac@parkway.sg
Web: www.parkwayhealth.com

Parkway Group Healthcare (ParkwayHealth), one of Asia's leading healthcare providers, is committed to bringing customers high-quality service and state-of-the-art facilities. The group's three hospitals are the first private hospitals in the Asia Pacific region to achieve ISO 9002 international quality certification. They have collectively performed one of the largest numbers of cardiac surgeries and neurosurgeries in the region's private healthcare sector.

With a reputation for excellence, ParkwayHealth's clinical programs are supported by 1,400 accredited medical specialists in heart and vascular medicine, neuroscience, oncology, musculoskeletal medicine, transplant and cellular therapy, women's and children's health, chronic disease management, and surgery.

Along with a comprehensive range of specialized tertiary healthcare services under one roof, ParkwayHealth also boasts several centers of excellence in specialties that include cardiology, andrology, urology, and oncology (see Gleneagles Hospital and Mount Elizabeth Hospital, below). The **International Patient Assistance Centre** operates a 24-hour hotline and serves as a one-stop service center to help international patients access specialist expertise, receive personalized patient care, and utilize cutting-edge technology at all ParkwayHealth hospitals in Singapore.

Member institutions include **East Shore Hospital*, Gleneagles Hospital*, and Mount Elizabeth Hospital*.** (* JCI-accredited.)

Services Provided for International Patients

✦ Appointment scheduling

✦ Flight arrangements and extensions

✦ Accommodations arrangement (hotel or service apartment)

✦ Visa arrangements and extensions

✦ Cost estimates and medical financial counseling

✦ Airport pickup by ambulance or limousine

✦ Medical referrals

✦ Language interpretation

✦ Special dietary and religious arrangements

✦ Arrangements for local sightseeing tours

✦ Evacuation and repatriation assistance

Feature Story

Hospital Care in Singapore Now Available to American Patients at Pre-Negotiated, In-Network Rates Far Lower than Comparable Services in the US (adapted press release, April 17, 2008)

Three hospitals operated by ParkwayHealth have become the first medical institutions in Singapore to join a US-based healthcare network and will treat American patients at pre-negotiated, in-network rates that are dramatically lower than those typically charged at US hospitals.

Clients of South Carolina–based Companion Global Healthcare, Inc. now have the option of traveling to Singapore's Mount Elizabeth, Gleneagles, or East Shore hospitals for a wide range of medical and surgical services, including joint replacement, open-heart and cardiology surgery, and invasive cancer treatment.

"This marks a significant milestone in the global reach of Singapore's healthcare," said Dr. Jason Yap, director of healthcare services for the Singapore Tourism Board. "Singapore has long been the leading medical hub and healthcare destination of choice in Asia. It is therefore not unexpected that Americans would also seek to avail themselves of high-quality healthcare in Singapore's safe and stable environment." More than 410,000 visitors traveled to Singapore for medical services in 2006.

"The addition of ParkwayHealth in Singapore means our individual clients and employer groups have more outstanding options for obtaining fully credentialed medical care at affordable, all-inclusive prices," said David Boucher, Companion Global Healthcare's assistant vice president of healthcare services.

Through Companion Global Healthcare's network, the more than

1 million members of Blue Cross Blue Shield of South Carolina and BlueChoice HealthPlan of South Carolina have access to Parkway-Health's three Singapore hospitals at preferred rates. The company provides a single launch point for appointments, travel services, case management, and followup care in the US. Companion Global Health-care is available to contract with insurance companies and employer groups that wish to include an overseas option in their benefit plans; it also serves the uninsured.

East Shore Hospital

321 Joo Chiat Place
SINGAPORE 427990
Tel: 65 6735.5000 (24-hour hotline)
Fax: 65 6345.4966
Email: ipac@parkway.sg
Web: www.eastshore.com.sg

East Shore Hospital is a 123-bed general and acute-care hospital offering services from general medicine to several specializations, such as surgery, pediatrics, and obstetrics and gynecology. Ancillary services include radiology, imaging, and rehabilitation therapy. East Shore Hospital received JCI accreditation in November 2007.

Gleneagles Hospital

6A Napier Road
SINGAPORE 258500
Tel: 65 6735.5000 (24-hour hotline)
Fax: 65 6475.1832
Email: ipac@parkway.sg
Web: www.gleneagles.com.sg

Established in 1957 and purchased by Parkway Group Health-care (now ParkwayHealth) in 1987, the JCI-accredited Gleneagles Hospital is a 380-bed, private, tertiary, acute-care facility. It has forged partnerships with Johns Hopkins Hospital (US) and Thames Valley Hospital (UK). With 280 specialists on staff, the hospital is a regional leader and referral center for the care and treatment of liver, cancer, and cardiac patients. It is also the first in Southeast Asia to use a robotic surgiscope for neurosurgery, spinal surgery, and ear, nose, and throat surgeries.

ParkwayHealth set up the **Asian Centre for Liver Diseases and Transplantation (ACLDT)** at Gleneagles Hospital in 1994. ACLDT is the first private center in Asia dedicated to treating all types of liver disease, including liver cancer, hepatitis, alcoholic cirrhosis, and pediatric liver disease. ACLDT has developed a highly successful transplant program in which a diseased liver is replaced with part of a liver from a healthy living donor. For patients with end-stage liver disease, this provides an alternative to waiting, sometimes indefinitely, for a suitable cadaveric donor.

In 2006 ParkwayHealth set up Asia's first dedicated liver intensive care unit. The new **Parkway Liver Centre,** together with ACLDT, provides fully integrated, comprehensive care supported by a team of multidisciplinary professionals, further enhancing Gleneagles Hospital's reputation as the region's leading facility for treatment of liver disease.

The **Parkway Cancer Centre (PCC)** is one of Asia's leading centers for cancer treatment. Led by a multidisciplinary team, the center provides comprehensive facilities for treating a wide range of cancers and optimizing patients' chances of recovery. PCC was first in Asia to utilize TomoTherapy, one of the latest radiation treatment systems, which precisely and painlessly delivers measured doses of radiation to the tumor and minimizes the exposure of healthy tissue.

PCC's other cutting-edge technologies include intensity modulated radiation therapy for tumors occurring very close to a critical organ; external radiation therapy; radiosurgery or stereotactic radiotherapy for tumors in the head and upper neck; and brachytherapy for cancers of the cervix, lung, esophagus, bile ducts, nose, and throat.

Specialties

✦ Cancer, cardiology, cardiothoracic and vascular surgery, gastroenterology and hepatology, hematology, lithotripsy, living donor liver transplant, liver diseases and transplantation, neuroscience, oral and maxillofacial surgery, neonatology, obstetrics and gynecology, ophthalmology, orthopedics, pediatrics, sports and exercise medicine, and urology

Achievements

✦ JCI accreditation in May 2006

✦ World's first living donor liver transplant, performed in the UK by doctors from Gleneagles Hospital in 1993

✦ Southeast Asia's first living donor liver transplant and living donor pediatric liver transplant

✦ Asia's first laparoscopic-assisted ventricular peritoneal placement in a newborn

✦ Southeast Asia's first delivery of sextuplets

Feature Story

I Got My Life (and Knee) Back in Singapore

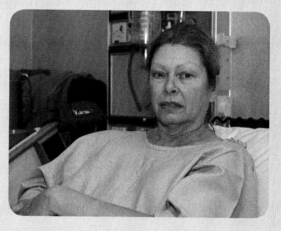

In 2003 Nancy fell after missing a step in her sunken living room, and she underwent arthroscopic surgery two months later to mend the badly torn cartilage in her knee—but that was not the end of the problem. "In 2006 my knee grew really painful, and it locked and swelled up a lot. By the summer of 2007, it was unbearable. The lower part of my leg was bent outwards," relates Nancy.

Her US doctors recommended a total knee replacement. However, without any medical insurance, the cost of surgery would set her back more than she felt she could afford. Nancy decided to consider treatment outside of the US and turned to Med Journeys (see the "Health Travel Agents" section), a US-based medical tourism company she found on the Internet.

What ultimately "sealed the deal" was the credentials of the surgeon that Med Journeys had identified: Dr. Ang Kian Chuan, consulting knee and shoulder surgeon at Singapore's Gleneagles Hospital. In June 2008, Nancy touched down in Singapore and was soon at the hospital for an x-ray of her knee.

The prior x-rays Nancy had sent to Dr. Ang indicated a "knock-knee" deformity: her tibia (shin bone) had turned outward about 30 degrees in relation to her femur (thigh bone). Concerns with joint replacement include misalignment, loosening, and longevity of the implant or prosthesis—and with a severe deformity or bone loss, exact alignment and orientation become even more important. "Nancy is still young, so to get her knee implant nice and straight, I decided on computer-navigated surgery to improve accuracy and get it as perfectly aligned as possible," says Dr. Ang.

Three days after her two-and-a-half-hour surgery, under the close watch of a physiotherapist, Nancy was out of bed and walking. She recalls, "I was amazed. The pain I had been suffering from for so long was gone." Nancy was discharged after five days.

"Dollar for dollar, it was really affordable, yet the quality of health-care here is up to world-class standards. The nursing care was excellent, and Dr. Ang was ever so patient. He made me feel assured and confident, because I could tell he knew what he was talking about," declares Nancy, who is also a registered nurse. "I used to get up in the morning, cry, and be miserable. My life was taken away, but thanks to Dr. Ang, I have it back, and of course, my knee too."

Mount Elizabeth Hospital

3 Mount Elizabeth
SINGAPORE 228510
Tel: 65 6737.2666 (24-hour hotline)
Fax: 65 6737.1189
Email: ipac@parkway.sg
Web: www.mountelizabeth.com.sg

Mount Elizabeth Hospital (MEH) is a private, tertiary, acute-care hospital with 505 beds. MEH has performed the most cardiac surgeries and neurosurgeries in the private sector in the region. It is also known for hematology, stem cell transplantation, PET/CT scanning, and robotic surgery.

The hospital's **Haematology and Stem Cell Transplant Centre** specializes in blood disorders, such as leukemia, thalassemia, and sickle cell anemia, as well as advanced cancers, such as those of the kidney, pancreas, and ovary. It is the first facility in Southeast Asia to offer cutting-edge stem cell transplant therapy for life-threatening cancers unresponsive to conventional treatments. This therapy improves the acute leukemia cure rate in adults from 20 percent to 80 percent and lowers the risk of death from treatment from 20 percent to 5 percent.

Specialties

✦ Cancer, cardiology and cardiothoracic surgery, hematology and stem cell transplant, LASIK, obstetrics and gynecology, neonatal intensive care, radiology and diagnostics, and diseases of the liver and digestive tract

Achievements

+ JCI accreditation in June 2006

+ World's first unrelated blood stem cell transplant and unrelated umbilical cord blood stem cell transplant for thalassemia major

+ Asia's first cardiomyoplasty and transmyocardial revascularization with the heart laser

+ Singapore's first private hospital to offer butler and concierge services to patients

+ Singapore's first PET/CT scanner

+ Southeast Asia's first minimally invasive robotic surgery using the four-arm Da Vinci Surgical System

+ Singapore's first private hospital to perform artificial corneal implantation

+ Singapore's first laparoscopic hernia repair

+ Singapore's first abdominal aortic aneurysm stenting

+ Singapore's first fibroid embolization

+ Singapore's first vertebroplasty

Feature Story

The Eagle Has Mended

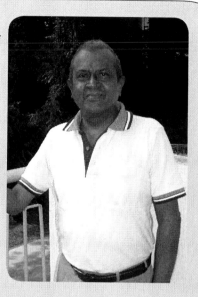

In 2005 58-year-old Denzil Gunaratne's life was rocked when an ultrasound examination of his liver revealed a tumor, which a biopsy confirmed to be malignant. After an extensive search, Denzil arrived in Singapore to consult with Dr. Tan Kai Chah, head of the Asian Centre for Liver Diseases and Transplantation at Gleneagles Hospital. Dr. Tan explains, "Examinations done on Denzil revealed that he had liver cirrhosis, where his liver tissue had hardened, and he also had liver cancer. Unfortunately, there is no treatment that can treat them both together except a liver transplant."

Widely esteemed as one of the world's best liver surgeons and a pioneer of living donor liver transplantation, Dr. Tan has performed more than 700 liver transplants, with approximately 150 involving live donors. This procedure is possible because as little as 30 percent of a liver is adequate to sustain normal function. For a living donor transplant, surgeons harvest 50 percent of the donor's liver; in two months, the organ will have grown back to its original size.

Having no relatives who could serve as a donor, Denzil turned to a good friend, but doctors in Singapore found that the friend's organ was a fatty liver and therefore unsuitable. Meanwhile, Denzil's wife had begun a search of her own, and when she spoke to a Buddhist monk at the temple she visits regularly, he offered to donate his liver. The selfless monk, 27-year-old Rev. Ariyawansha Thero, wanted absolutely nothing in return—and, even more amazingly, he had previously donated a kidney to someone else.

In July 2007, Denzil brought Rev. Thero to Singapore, where Dr. Tan and his team verified the suitability of the monk's liver. An independent medical ethics committee conducted an assessment to determine whether the donor was of sound mind with a stable financial standing, and whether there was any exchange of money in the arrangement. Following this assessment, Denzil's eight-hour transplant went ahead without a glitch.

Dr. Tan emphasizes, "Liver transplantation is not a one-man show. A full team is needed, and at Gleneagles Hospital, we are fortunate to have such a team, which includes an intensivist, cardiologist, psychiatrist, anesthetist, infectious disease specialist, renal physician, and specialist nurses who are trained to look after liver patients."

Denzil is all praise for the efficiency and systematic way of doing things that he observed in Singapore. This mended legal eagle now looks set to enjoy many more days in court.

Raffles Medical Group

Raffles International Patients Centre
Raffles Hospital
585 North Bridge Road
SINGAPORE 188770
Tel: 65 6311.1666
Fax: 65 6311.2333
Email: enquiries@raffleshospital.com
Web: www.rafflesmedical.com

Raffles Medical Group (RMG), one of Singapore's largest private healthcare providers, is an extensive network of 60 Raffles Medical Clinics island-wide and a flagship facility, Raffles Hospital. Raffles Health, a preventive care unit, offers a full range of nutraceuticals, supplements, vitamins, and medical diagnostic equipment.

Raffles Hospital is a full-service private hospital offering a full complement of specialist services combined with advanced medical technology in well-equipped diagnostic and treatment facilities. Its staff and visiting consultants work as a team in a holistic approach to patient care. Patients have access to a large number of specialists and enjoy the quality assurance of peer-reviewed and medically audited services. The hospital also adheres to a fixed and transparent fee schedule.

Raffles Hospital's well-appointed inpatient rooms are outfitted to the standards of a five-star hotel, with an array of suites and single-, double-, four-, and six-bed rooms for patients to choose from. Located in the heart of the city and a 20-minute drive from Changi International Airport, the hospital is conveniently close to shopping centers, restaurants, and food stores.

Specialties

✦ Cardiology, cardiothoracic surgery, dentistry and dental surgery, dermatology, endocrinology, gastroenterology, geriatric medicine, hand surgery, hepatology, internal medicine, medical oncology, neurology, neurosurgery, obstetrics and gynecology, ophthalmology, orthopedic surgery, pediatric medicine, pathology, plastic and reconstructive surgery, renal medicine, respiratory medicine, rheumatology, sports medicine, urology, and surgery of the ear, nose, and throat

Services Provided for International Patients

✦ Appointment scheduling

✦ Travel planning

✦ Airport pickup and transportation

✦ Assistance with admissions and discharge

✦ Medical referrals

✦ Language interpretation and secretarial services

✦ Concierge services

✦ Goods and Services Tax refund

✦ Evacuation and repatriation assistance

Achievements

✦ Group-wide ISO 9001:2000 certification

✦ Successful separation surgery of Korean conjoined twins in 2003

Feature Story

A Balloon Up My Nose

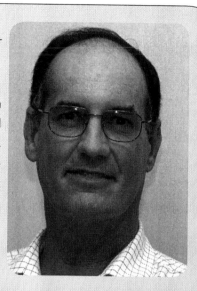

"For eight years, 24/7, 365 days a year, I had to endure constant head and face pains, plugged-up ears, nose congestion, colds, and vertigo," exclaims 49-year-old Scott Drawe, in his distinctive Texas accent. Although the retired petroleum engineer had previously visited a top US hospital in 2003, extensive testing — which cost about US$20,000 — had only managed to come up with a diagnosis of "asthma-like symptoms."

In 2006 Scott had a serious motorcycle accident in Vietnam and required extensive treatment for his facial injuries. International SOS (see the "Health Travel Agents" section) evacuated him to Singapore's Raffles Hospital, where he eventually made a full recovery. In a bizarre way, that episode led to another good result: at a followup check several months later, Scott contacted the hospital's International Patients Centre to see a specialist about his nasal problem.

Scott met with Dr. Stephen Lee, a consulting ear, nose, and throat surgeon and senior partner at Raffles Hospital. A CT scan confirmed Dr. Lee's initial suspicions that Scott had sinusitis, an inflammation of the sinus lining. "The efficiency at Raffles was alien to me. Here, you don't have to wait three months to see a specialist or three hours to have a scan like in the US," shares Scott, who cited Dr. Lee's systematic approach and competence as being "very assuring."

Dr. Lee outlines, "Many patients just have a sinus issue, but with

Scott, besides narrowed sinuses, his nasal septum (cartilage and bony wall separating the nostrils) was deviated (possibly from birth) to one side, which was also obstructing his airways and causing him pressure symptoms and constant headaches."

Scott agreed to treatment with a relatively new procedure known as balloon sinuplasty. Employing technology garnered from cardiac balloon angioplasty, this technique involves putting a wire through a guide catheter (tubing) at the narrowed pathway, railroading a deflated balloon to that narrowed point, and pumping up the balloon until it becomes firm and rigid, thus opening up that sinus area. The procedure typically takes just under an hour.

Dr. Lee has utilized balloon sinuplasty on more than 100 sinuses and trains surgeons from throughout Asia in this method. He enthuses, "What is great about this technique is that there is little bleeding, and patients regain full ability to breathe after surgery. Downtime is short, and patients can get back to work very quickly."

Indeed, by the next day, Scott was up and in high spirits. He relates, "I was breathing freely, something I had not been able to do for the past eight years. I could actually feel air up my nose. It was amazing."

SINGAPORE HEALTH SERVICES

SingHealth International Medical Services
Singapore General Hospital
Block 6, Level 1, Outram Road
SINGAPORE 169608
Tel: 65 6326.5656
Fax: 65 6326.5900
Email: ims@singhealth.com.sg
Web: www.singhealth.com.sg

Singapore Health Services (SingHealth) is Singapore's largest group of healthcare institutions, with three hospitals, five national specialty centers, and a network of primary care clinics. Each member of the group makes a unique contribution to the integrated organization. Under the SingHealth umbrella, these facilities jointly provide a multidisciplinary and multi-institutional approach to high-quality medical service.

Supported by a strong teaching tradition and a wide spectrum of 42 clinical specialties, SingHealth is also an ideal training ground for the continuing development of medical personnel. SingHealth measures itself against international standards to ensure clinical excellence and continually evolves to stay at the leading edge of medicine. Its medical breakthroughs have helped to put Singapore on the global healthcare map and have also translated into improved treatment techniques.

SingHealth's **International Medical Services** team acts as a one-stop service center, providing a wide spectrum of services to international patients and their families at the group's various healthcare facilities.

Member institutions serving international patients include **Changi General Hospital*, KK Women's and Children's**

Hospital*, Singapore General Hospital*, National Cancer Centre Singapore, National Dental Centre, National Heart Centre Singapore*, National Neuroscience Institute, and **Singapore National Eye Centre.** (* JCI-accredited.)

Services Provided for International Patients

✦ Appointment and referral scheduling

✦ Arrangements for accommodations

✦ Airport pickup and transportation

✦ Admission assistance

✦ Language interpretation

✦ Private nursing

✦ Business center

✦ Concierge services

✦ Evacuation and repatriation assistance

Changi General Hospital

2 Simei Street 3
SINGAPORE 529889
Tel: 65 6260.3725
Fax: 65 6850.2905
Email: international@cgh.com.sg
Web: www.cgh.com.sg

Changi General Hospital (CGH) offers a comprehensive range of medical, surgical, and paramedical services, as well as a medical center for international travelers. A mere ten minutes from

Changi International Airport, CGH is an emerging expert in gastroenterology, dermatology, obstructive sleep apnea, sports medicine, prostate management, male impotence, urinary incontinence, cartilage transplant, arthroscopy, one-stop breast care, and multiphasic health screening. The hospital is well equipped with modern technology, such as MRI, spiral CT, and cardiac catheterization systems.

Specialties

✦ Cardiology, dermatology, otolaryngology, ophthalmology, gastroenterology, geriatric medicine, multiphasic health screening, neurology and neurosurgery, obstetrics and gynecology, oral and maxillofacial surgery, orthopedic surgery, radiology, rehabilitative medicine, sports medicine, and urology

Achievements

✦ JCI accreditation in June 2005

✦ ISO 9002:1994, ISO 14000, and ISO 9001:2000 certifications

✦ Asian Hospital Management Award

KK Women's and Children's Hospital

100 Bukit Timah Road
SINGAPORE 229899
Tel: 65 6394.8888 (24-hour hotline)
Fax: 65 6293.7933
Email: international@kkh.com.sg
Web: www.kkh.com.sg

KK Women's and Children's Hospital (KKH) is the largest facility in Singapore providing specialized care for women, babies, and children. It is a major tertiary referral center for high-risk obstetrics, gynecological oncology, urogynecology, neonatology, pediatrics, pediatric bone marrow transplant, and pediatric open-heart surgery.

KKH is also Singapore's only integrated women's and children's hospital. **KK Women's Hospital** has been devoted to women's healthcare for 80 years and has several subspecialty units, including sports medicine and plastic, reconstructive, and aesthetic surgery. **KK Children's Hospital** is dedicated to healing and fighting illnesses in children up to 16 years old, offering a wide range of pediatric medical and surgical services.

KKH's centers of excellence include

✦ **KK Breast Centre,** a one-stop facility housing Singapore's first state-of-the-art breast imaging center, which combines digital mammography, breast ultrasonography, surgical consultation, minimally invasive biopsy, and other procedures under one roof and with quick turnaround. The Breast Imaging Unit is the world's first to use FDA-approved computed radiography (CR) technology for mammography combined with computer-aided detection (CAD). This digital form of mammography is superior to traditional film mammography and enables more cancers to be detected earlier.

✢ **KK Minimally Invasive Surgery Centre,** specialized in gynecology with expertise in endoscopic surgery. The center provides state-of-the-art facilities for outpatient and inpatient procedures. The latest technology at KK Women's Hospital, the ExAblate 2000, uses MRI to focus ultrasound waves for nonsurgical treatment of uterine fibroids.

✢ **Cleft and Craniofacial Centre,** Singapore's only dedicated, comprehensive craniofacial service. Patients with craniofacial disorders, including those with jaw injuries, are usually referred to the center for assessment and treatment.

✢ **Children's Cancer Centre,** one of Southeast Asia's largest, treating 70 percent of childhood cancers in Singapore, with a growing number of regional referrals. Its team of six pediatric oncologists, a pediatric neurosurgeon, and a pediatric oncology surgeon is assisted in caring for the center's patients by specially trained pediatric nurses and paramedical personnel.

Specialties

KK Women's Hospital:

✢ Aesthetic and reconstructive surgery, breast health, maternal fetal medicine, general obstetrics and gynecology, gynecological oncology, menopause, minimally invasive surgery, orthopedic surgery, otolaryngology, reproductive medicine, and urogynecology

KK Children's Hospital:

✦ Cardiology, endocrinology, gastroenterology, genetics, hematology and oncology, infectious diseases, neonatology, nephrology, neurology, respiratory medicine, rheumatology, immunology and allergy, cardiothoracic surgery, dental surgery, neurosurgery, ophthalmology, orthopedic surgery, otolaryngology, and plastic and reconstructive surgery

Achievements

✦ JCI accreditation in December 2005

✦ Asia's first delivery of a gamete intrafallopian transfer (GIFT) baby

✦ Asia's first digital colposcopy system for screening cervical cancer

✦ Asia's first endoanal pull-through procedure for Hirschsprung's disease

✦ Southeast Asia's first microwave endometrial ablation procedure to treat heavy menstruation

✦ Southeast Asia's first hospital to offer the tension-free vaginal tape operation for urinary incontinence

✦ Singapore's first laparoscopic-assisted vaginal hysterectomy

✦ Singapore's first blood transfusion for a baby in the womb

✦ Introduced a new laser-assisted hatching technique to boost pregnancy rates for IVF

Feature Story

MR-Guided Focused Ultrasound Ablation for Uterine Fibroids

Patricia, a Hong Kong resident, was diagnosed with hysteromyoma, also known as uterine fibroids, in 2004. She was not too concerned initially, given the condition's commonality. But when her symptoms took a turn for the worse in early 2007, she had no choice but to seek treatment.

While she was researching various treatments on the Internet, a particular report caught her eye: MR-guided focused ultrasound ablation (MRgFUS), a revolutionary, noninvasive, painless procedure for removing uterine fibroids, offered by KK Women's and Children's Hospital in Singapore. MRgFUS combines a high-intensity focused ultrasound beam, which heats and destroys the targeted fibroid tissue, with MRI, which visualizes the anatomy to monitor the beam's effect in real time.

Patricia immediately emailed an inquiry to KKH. She soon received a detailed response from Professor David Stringer, head and senior consultant of the Department of Diagnostic Imaging. Prof. Stringer explained that because uterine fibroids vary in location and size, and because the texture of the uterus varies, not all fibroids can be successfully removed with this treatment. He suggested that Patricia undergo an MRI scan before deciding whether to proceed with MRgFUS. Upon that advice, she made an appointment for a thorough examination at KKH.

In April 2007, Patricia flew to Singapore. After her MRI, she decided to proceed with the MRgFUS procedure. She recalls thinking, "This is a non-traumatic and risk-free procedure. Why not give it a try and give myself a chance? Even if it fails, I can still try other treatments."

During the procedure, Patricia had to lie flat and maintain the same position for almost four hours. Along with radiologists and nurses, a physiotherapist was present to monitor Patricia for any potential deep vein thrombosis (DVT) from spending such a lengthy time in a fixed position. Despite her slight discomfort, Patricia was moved by the care of the attentive and friendly staff, who ensured that all of her needs were met.

After her treatment, Patricia returned to Hong Kong, where the KKH doctors and nurses called her regularly to check on her recovery. She was impressed by such devoted attention, thoughtfulness, and personalized care, which she says are unheard of in the UK and Hong Kong.

Singapore General Hospital

International Medical Service
Block 6, Level 1, Outram Road
SINGAPORE 169608
Tel: 65 6326.5656
Fax: 65 6326.5900
Email: ims@sgh.com.sg
Web: www.sgh.com.sg

Established in 1821, Singapore General Hospital (SGH) is Singapore's oldest and largest acute-care, tertiary hospital. SGH is the national referral center for plastic surgery and burns, renal medicine, nuclear medicine, pathology, and hematology. The hospital provides multidisciplinary medical care, and its patients have ready access to more than 30 clinical specialties.

SGH is committed to achieving excellence in its "three pillars": service, teaching, and research. It has been a pioneer in medical education since Singapore's first medical and nursing schools were established in the early 1900s. With the emergence of specialty departments, the hospital began to play a more prominent role in postgraduate medical education and is now the principal training ground for specialists. Four specialty centers are located within the SGH compound: the **National Cancer Centre, National Dental Centre, National Heart Centre Singapore,** and **Singapore National Eye Centre.**

Specialties

+ Colorectal surgery, dermatology, diagnostic radiology, endocrinology, gastroenterology, geriatric medicine, hematology, hand surgery, internal medicine, neonatal and developmental medicine, neurology, neurosurgery, nuclear medicine and PET, obstetrics and gynecology, orthopedic surgery, pathology, rehabilitative medicine, renal medicine, respiratory and critical care medicine, rheumatology and immunology, urology, plastic surgery, reconstructive surgery, aesthetic surgery, and surgery of the ear, nose, and throat

Achievements

+ Asia's largest teaching hospital to attain JCI accreditation, in July 2005
+ College of American Pathologists accreditation
+ Southeast Asia's first cochlear implant surgery
+ Singapore's first heart transplant

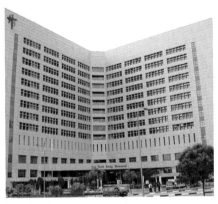

Tan Tock Seng Hospital

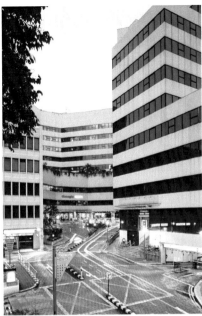

ParkwayHealth's Gleneagles Hospital

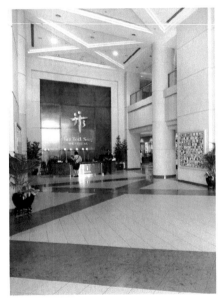

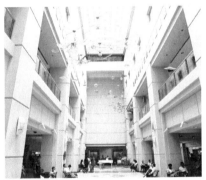

Sky Garden at Tan Tock Seng Hospital

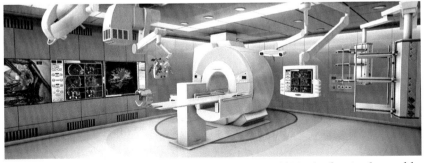

Located at Singapore General Hospital, the BrainSUITE is the first in the world

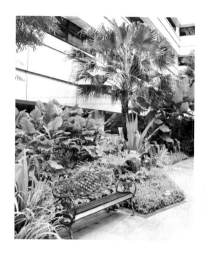

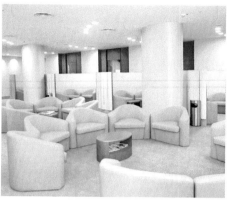

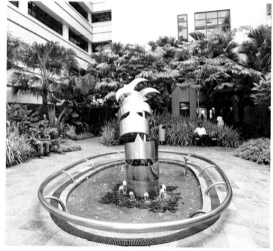

Lush gardens, soothing waterfalls, and private sanctuaries await you at Singapore General Hospital

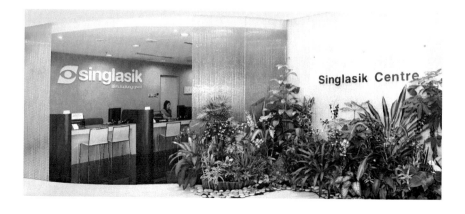

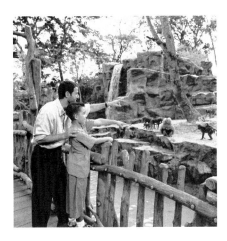

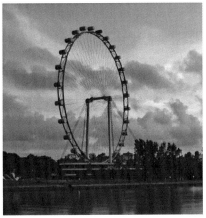

From elaborate
theme parks to
award-winning zoos
and parks, Singapore
offers something
for everybody

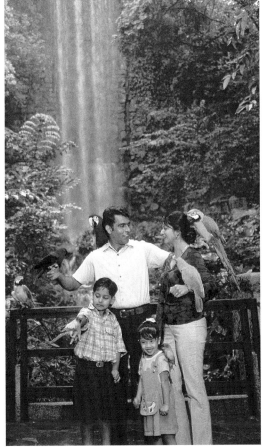

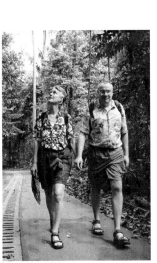

Biopolis,
Asia's leading
biomedical
research and
development hub

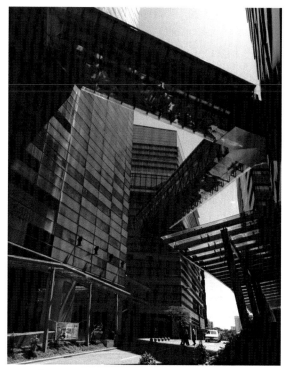

Biopolis

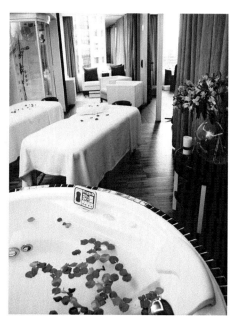

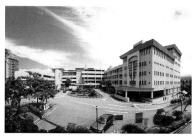

Mount Alvernia Hospital

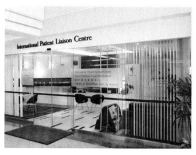

Pacific Healthcare Group's Wellness
Lounge, a premier medical aesthetics spa

International Patient Liaison Centre

✤ Asia's first successful pregnancy using surgical sperm retrieval

✤ Asia's first percutaneous endoscopic gall bladder removal

✤ Southeast Asia's first hospital to provide catheter ablation

✤ Asia's first virtual reality surgery for tumor removal

✤ Asia's first human bilateral fetal brain cell transplant for Parkinson's disease

✤ Singapore's first lung transplant

✤ Successful separation of a pair of craniopagus (fused heads) conjoined twins from Nepal

✤ World's first forearm attachment to shoulder blade

Feature Story

An Indian Patient Walks Tall Again

Mitta Narayan Kuppuswami is a sprightly 81-year-old who walks confidently without any help — but this is a far cry from his condition three years ago, when the retired Indian national could barely keep his legs straight. "He was in so much pain, he had to pull up his legs and keep his knees bent to mitigate the acute pain. Every day, he would be popping pain killers," recalls his son, Raj. The family deliberated between Singapore and the US for Mr. Mitta's operation and rehabilitation.

"In terms of the quality and experience of surgeons, India is probably as good, and we could have just had the surgeries there. But in terms of hospital care and post-operative care, we felt Singapore has the leading edge," explains Raj. "My father likes to get involved in what's happening. He likes to sit down and really talk to the doctor, to understand what's to be done for him. In India, patients just don't get that kind of personal attention from their doctors, because the sheer volume of patients makes that impossible."

The turning point in the senior Mitta's life came when father and son sought help from Dr. Amit Mitra, a senior consultant in the Department of Orthopaedics at Singapore General Hospital. Dr. Mitra recalls, "When the patient first came to me, he was barely able to walk. I could see he was suffering, and I told him both his knees must be replaced. They had become grossly deformed from arthritis."

The surgeon took a standard approach with a 4-inch (10-centimeter) incision. The damaged part of the joint was removed, the surfaces of the bones were reshaped to hold a metal joint, and the artificial joint was then attached to the thigh bone, shin, and kneecap with cement. The entire process took about two hours, after which Mr. Mitta rested in bed for a day before beginning rehabilitative physiotherapy. "The very next day, we encourage the patient to start walking. It is very painful, of course, but the goal is to get the muscles to regain strength, so that the leg can regain its range of movement," explains Dr. Mitra.

Knee joint replacements are commonly performed at SGH, about 1,500 cases each year. Each surgery costs SGD3,500–10,000. The younger Mitta is effusive in his praise for his father's treatment experience. "The doctors and hospital did an outstanding job. My father and I were extremely happy with everything, from the doctor's professionalism to the aftercare services!"

National Cancer Centre Singapore

11 Hospital Drive
SINGAPORE 169610
Tel: 65 6236.9433
Fax: 65 6536.0611
Email: foreign_patient@nccs.com.sg
Web: www.nccs.com.sg

The National Cancer Centre Singapore (NCCS) is a national and regional center dedicated to the prevention and treatment of cancers, including thoracic, hepatobiliary (liver and bile ducts), pancreatic, head, and neck cancers. As a one-stop specialist center housing Singapore's largest pool of oncologists, NCCS uses advanced equipment and employs the latest therapies, including mini-transplants and targeted therapies that maximize outcomes and minimize undesirable side effects. It sees over 50 percent of the cancer patients in Singapore.

Physically and operationally designed to provide integrated, holistic, patient-centered services, the center promotes cross-consultation among oncologists of different specialties. Patients can therefore be assessed by more than one specialist during the same visit. NCCS also conducts clinical and basic research and develops public cancer education programs directed toward prevention and treatment.

National Heart Centre Singapore

Mistri Wing
17 Third Hospital Avenue
SINGAPORE 168752
Tel: 65 6236.7438
Fax: 65 6323.0663
Email: gps@nhc.com.sg
Web: www.nhc.com.sg

The National Heart Centre Singapore (NHC) is the national referral center for cardiovascular disease. NHC provides comprehensive preventive, diagnostic, therapeutic, and rehabilitative cardiac services to local and overseas patients. Its multidisciplinary team carries out approximately 75,000 cardiac investigative procedures and over 6,000 heart operations annually.

In addition to diagnostic and therapeutic cardiac services, NHC provides structured programs in cardiovascular rehabilitative and preventive cardiology to enhance the recovery process. The center's survival rate for heart transplants compares favorably with standards established in other international institutions. NHC's lung transplantation program, started in 1999, offers hope for some patients who have final-stage lung disease.

Achievements

✦ JCI accreditation in October 2005

✦ Air repatriation of a German myocarditis patient

✦ Asia Pacific region's first implantation of a percutaneous left atrial appendage transcatheter occlusion device, which halves the risk of stroke

✦ Asia's first cardiac arrhythmia surgery

Feature Story

Stem Cell Research Breakthrough for Treating Heart Failure

Stem cell researchers and clinicians at Singapore's National Heart Centre have made an important breakthrough. Studies have revealed that heart-like cells, generated from an adult patient's own stem cells and then transplanted into the patient's heart, contribute to increasing the ailing heart's pumping force. This clinical research — the first of its kind in the world — shows that these stem cells converted into heart-like cells before transplant are more effective than transplanting whole stem cells directly, which is currently the most widely used cell therapy for heart failure.

After a heart attack, many patients sustain irreversible cardiac injury, leading to heart failure and symptoms of breathlessness. For patients with severely damaged hearts, a whole-organ heart transplant is sometimes the only hope, but finding a donor is a tremendous challenge.

Through processes developed at NHC, the stem cells of a patient with heart failure can potentially be harvested and processed in a lab for a few weeks to optimize them, and then the patient's own converted heart-like cells can be transplanted back into the heart to help repair or "heal" it. This may alleviate symptoms and delay the need for a whole-organ transplant. Because the process uses the patient's own cells, immunosuppressants to prevent rejection are unnecessary.

This study, in its sixth year, has involved the stem cells of 43 patients undergoing bypass surgery; a patent has been filed for the isolation and expansion procedures producing the heart-like cells. In addition to improving pumping action, these cells have been found to be "smarter," as they are able to move themselves into areas of the heart that need them most. They also aid in preventing heart swelling, a detrimental and often irreversible process that makes treatment more difficult.

"It is an exciting time for NHC as our own scientists, working with clinicians, bring their own research, validated and tested, to benefit our patients," says Dr. Philip Wong, director of NHC's R&D Unit and a senior consultant in the Department of Cardiology. The cell therapy research program is in its final translational phase, and clinicians have been optimizing a nonsurgical method of delivering the cells to the heart.

National Neuroscience Institute

11 Jalan Tan Tock Seng
SINGAPORE 308433
Tel: 65 8128.8007
Fax: 65 6357.7103
Email: nni_secretariat@nni.com.sg
Web: www.nni.com.sg

The National Neuroscience Institute (NNI), a specialized center for the management and care of neurological disease, provides treatment for a broad range of illnesses that affect the brain, spine, nerves, and muscle. NNI is one of the few centers in Asia participating in international clinical trials for new medications, particularly for stroke treatment. It is the first facility in Southeast Asia to utilize the highly accurate 3-Tesla MRI scanner, which produces better neuroimaging for patients with stroke, epilepsy, and other neurological conditions.

In 2006 NNI collaborated with BrainLAB AG, a global leader in software-driven systems for targeted, less-invasive medical treatments, to establish the world's first state-of-the-art, digitally integrated neuroscience center. The five-suite facility sets a new standard for clinical results and overall cost-effectiveness in neurosurgery, otolaryngology, and orthopedic surgery. With real-time intra-operative MRI, CT, and advanced image-guided navigation systems, surgeons are able to monitor progress during operations and perform more complicated surgeries more quickly and with improved patient outcomes.

Singapore National Eye Centre

11 Third Hospital Avenue
Outram Road
SINGAPORE 168751
Tel: 65 6100.9393
Fax: 65 6222.9393
Email: ips@snec.com.sg
Web: www.snec.com.sg

The Singapore National Eye Centre (SNEC) spearheads and coordinates the national provision of specialized ophthalmologic services. With a staff of 450 medical, paramedical, and administrative personnel, SNEC is known for its high-quality, one-stop, personalized patient care. The center is also actively involved in clinical trials and research into the causes and treatment of major eye conditions, such as myopia and glaucoma. Thousands of ophthalmologists from neighboring countries and beyond have participated in SNEC's teaching courses and international meetings.

Specialties

✢ Cataract and comprehensive ophthalmology, corneal and external eye disease, glaucoma, neuro-ophthalmology, ocular inflammation and immunology, oculoplastic and aesthetic eye surgery, pediatric ophthalmology and strabismus correction, refractive surgery, and vitreoretinal surgery

---

Feature Story

"Tooth-in-Eye" Surgery

Eye surgeons at the Singapore National Eye Centre have successfully completed a revolutionary two-stage surgical procedure to restore a young blind man's sight. The patient, 19-year-old Luck Pewnual from Thailand, completely lost his sight in both eyes six years ago as a result of a rare allergic reaction. Thanks to his "tooth-in-eye" surgery at SNEC, believed to be the first operation of its kind in Southeast Asia, he is now able to see well.

The first stage of the surgery was performed in February 2004 and involved five separate procedures: opening one eye and removing the eyelids' entire inner surface, the corneal surface, and scar tissue from the allergic reaction; removing the cheek's inner mucosal lining and transplanting it onto the eye's new surface; removing a canine tooth and part of the adjacent bone and attached ligaments; fashioning a bolt-shaped structure from this tooth-bone complex to receive a plastic optical cylinder, which was cemented on; and implanting the tooth-bone-cylinder complex into his cheek to grow a new blood supply.

The second stage, performed in June 2004, involved two separate

---

procedures first: opening the cheek mucosal lining over the eye and making a circular opening in the cornea to receive the implant, while also removing the inner front contents of the eye (iris, lens, and anterior vitreous); then the living tooth-bone-cylinder complex was removed from the cheek, examined for viability, trimmed, and placed within the cornea, and the mucosal cheek lining was replaced over the implant. At the end of the procedure, light could once again enter the eye through the implanted cylinder.

Since the operation was completed, Luck has had minor eyelid surgery and a final surgical adjustment to the implant, and his vision has steadily improved. Luck has now attained 6/12 vision, which is enough to drive a car legally, and he also has excellent vision for reading.

Thomson Medical Centre

International Patient Centre
339 Thomson Road, Level 5
SINGAPORE 307677
Tel: 65 6250.1965 (24-hour hotline)
Fax: 65 6352.6551
Email: ipd@tmc-sin.com.sg
Web: www.thomsonmedical.com

Thomson Medical Centre (TMC) was established in 1979 as a hospital for women and children. It offers high-quality medical treatment and personalized patient care in a friendly, home-like environment. A 190-bed, acute-care, private hospital, TMC provides a comprehensive range of services with specialties in obstetrics, gynecology, and pediatrics.

The hospital offers fully integrated medical, surgical, therapeutic, diagnostic, and preventive healthcare services to ensure optimal management of childbirth. These services include specialist clinics, an x-ray and ultrasound center, a fetal assessment unit, a breast clinic, and a fertility center. TMC also provides programs in childbirth education, infant-care training, and confinement nanny service, as well as a hospital familiarization tour before childbirth.

Assisted reproductive services at **Thomson Fertility Centre (TFC)**, led by a team of experienced embryologists, give hope to couples who have little chance of conceiving naturally. IVF can be stressful, and anxiety can adversely affect the outcome, so the center simplifies its IVF program to minimize the complexities and reduce the pressure that couples may feel.

Since its inception, TFC has treated more than 4,000 infertile couples and achieved many local and international medical breakthroughs. The center delivered Singapore's first set of IVF triplets and Asia's first set of surviving IVF quadruplets. The world's first pair of twins from frozen eggs and frozen testicular sperm was conceived at TFC.

Specialties

✦ Obstetrics and gynecology, pediatrics, and fertility treatment

Services Provided for International Patients

✦ Appointment scheduling

✦ Flight reservations and confirmations

✦ Accommodations arrangement (hotel and service apartments)

✦ Financial counseling and cost estimation

✦ Visa arrangements and extensions

✦ Airport pickup and transportation

✦ Admission and discharge assistance

✦ Medical referrals

✦ Language interpretation

✦ Concierge services

Achievements

✦ Delivered its first baby from intracytoplasmic sperm injection (ICSI) in 1995

✦ Delivered its first baby from assisted-hatching treatment in 1999

Feature Story

World's First Births from Frozen Eggs and Frozen Testicular Sperm

The survival of frozen eggs is difficult to achieve, and so far only about 30 births from frozen eggs have been recorded worldwide. In a unique breakthrough, chief scientist Dr. Chia Choy May and her team at Thomson Fertility Clinic have achieved the world's first successful pregnancy from frozen eggs and frozen testicular sperm.

Dr. Chia explains: "The couple that came for the fertility treatment had a more complicated health history than usual. The husband had no sperm in the ejaculate, so we had to extract the sperm from the testes. The extracted sperm was frozen in preparation for an IVF/ICSI cycle.

"His wife went through IVF, and she had over 30 eggs at egg collection. Only eight eggs were injected, while the remaining eggs were frozen to prevent aging. Due to the patient's hyperstimulated condition, no embryo transfer was attempted.

"Five months later, the patient returned for a thaw cycle in which the frozen and thawed eggs were subjected to ICSI with the thawed testicular sperm. Although the patient did become pregnant, unfortunately the pregnancy ended in a miscarriage.

"The patient returned for a second thaw cycle six months later. Eighty percent of the remaining 12 frozen eggs survived. Two embryos resulting from ICSI of the frozen and thawed testicular sperm into the frozen and thawed eggs were transferred, and this culminated in the recent birth of a pair of healthy twins. The twins were of a good weight (more than 2 kilograms) and were successfully delivered by Cesarean section."

A spokesperson for Thomson Medical Centre says, "We are making constant breakthroughs at Thomson Fertility Clinic so as to offer hope and the best fertility solutions to couples who need help and intervention in conceiving. We are equally committed to giving our best efforts to support the government's fertility policy by searching out new techniques to help more couples conceive."

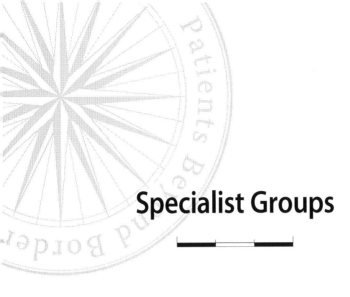

Specialist Groups

eMenders Medical Specialist Group

304 Orchard Road
#05-55A Lucky Plaza
SINGAPORE 238863
Tel: 65 6388.8939
Fax: 65 6835.7197
Email: info@emenders.com
Web: www.emenders.com

Based at Mount Elizabeth Medical Centre, eMenders is a group of more than 50 leading specialists covering more than 25 areas of medicine and dentistry. All eMenders specialists have international qualifications and additional international training, and most have held senior appointments at health and educational institutions. They have authored articles published in peer-reviewed journals and are regularly invited to speak at local and international conferences.

Patients can visit the eMenders Web site to find out about common problems and treatments for various medical conditions and to make inquiries and appointments with a medical or dental specialist. eMenders can also coordinate appointments for patients who would like to see several doctors from different specialty areas during their visit to Singapore.

Feature Story

A Breath of Relief

In 1974 casino dealer Michael Hornholtz was rolled into an operating room in California, expecting that the doctors would fix his broken nose and all would be well. But when the anesthesia wore off, he immediately knew something had gone wrong. "I had a torturous and intolerable pain at the site of the surgery. This was accompanied by extreme irritation of the membrane and floods of mucus, and the sensation that something was trapped in my nose," Michael recalls.

After repeated trials of medication, such as prescribed pain relievers and steroid spray, he became convinced that something serious was underlying his ongoing painful condition — but x-rays revealed only that his septum had been successfully corrected, and CT and MRI scans also failed to show anything conclusively.

Michael did some research and found out about a way to determine the exact nature of the problem through a minimally invasive examination using a microscopic camera; however, his doctors did not think that his condition warranted it. In 1996 a surgeon finally agreed to treat him, but the attempt was unsuccessful, as was another surgeon's attempt in 2003. Emotionally drained and financially strained, Michael nevertheless persevered for a solution.

He then came across Planet Hospital (see the "Health Travel Agents" section), a US-based organization that helps patients find the best and safest hospitals and surgeons around the world for their treatment needs. From the options, Michael decided to see Dr. Lau Chee Chong, a consultant ear, nose, and throat surgeon at Mount Elizabeth Medical Centre and part of the eMenders group of specialists.

In May 2007, Michael was met in Singapore by Planet Hospital's country manager. Michael relates, "He took care of everything, from my hotel reservations to accompanying me to, and providing transportation for, all my appointments. For a person undergoing such a difficult experience in a foreign country, this was invaluable."

About his doctor, he says, "Dr. Lau was very responsive and reassuring, and seemed to have a better understanding and a more positive approach towards my condition." Dr. Lau outlines Michael's chronic nasal problem: "What I saw was a lot of scar tissue in the anterior ethmoidal, an area where the nerves run. His septum had deviated to one side and was pressing against the lateral wall of the nose, a condition known as nasal neuralgia. This probably resulted when the doctors were trying to straighten his nose."

An hour-long operation cleared up the sinus infection and cleaned out the scar tissue left behind from his previous surgeries. Michael enthuses, "It became apparent that the trauma that had plagued me and controlled my life for so long was finally gone. Unbelievable!"

Island Orthopaedic Group

Mount Elizabeth:
3 Mount Elizabeth
#06-03 Mount Elizabeth Medical Centre
SINGAPORE 238510
Tel: 65 6737.5683
Fax: 65 6732.7290
Email: ioc_mte@iog.com.sg
Web: www.iog.com.sg

Gleneagles:
6 Napier Road
#02-16 Gleneagles Medical Centre
SINGAPORE 258499
Tel: 65 6474.5488
Fax: 65 6476.1697
Email: ioc_glen@iog.com.sg
Web: www.iog.com.sg

Established in 1995, Island Orthopaedic Group (IOG) is a private orthopedic practice with seven consultant orthopedic surgeons and a consultant sports physician. It provides specialized orthopedic and trauma care with subspecialties in knee and hip replacement, sports medicine, and injury and spinal surgery.

In addition to **Island Orthopaedic Consultants,** IOG's specialist practices include

✦**Island Spine and Scoliosis,** the spinal service division. It focuses on managing neck and back problems and offers detailed advice on the diagnosis, prognosis, and treatment options available. Spinal surgery is performed by its team of experienced surgeons trained in the management of complex spinal conditions and using the latest surgical techniques and equipment.

+ **Island Sports Medicine and Surgery,** made up of trained orthopedic sports surgeons with each surgeon specializing in specific areas of interest.

+ **SportsMed Central,** providing general sports medicine services to manage sports- and exercise-related injuries and enhance overall health and performance in sports. Clinical services include diagnosis and nonsurgical management of sports injuries, extracorporeal shock wave therapy (ESWT), preventive sport-medical screening, weight management, sports nutrition, and performance enhancement. SportsMed Central is affiliated with the ATOS Klinik in Heidelberg.

SportsMed Central is equipped with the state-of-the-art Dornier Epos Ultra to provide ultrasound-guided ESWT for treatment of various painful conditions, including heel pain (plantar fasciitis), tennis elbow, golfer's elbow, patellar tendonitis (jumper's knee), Achilles tendonitis, calcific tendonitis of the shoulder, and other injuries.

Specialist Dental Group

Mount Elizabeth Medical Centre
3 Mount Elizabeth #08-08
SINGAPORE 228510
Tel: 65 6734.9393
Fax: 65 6733.6032
Email: info@specialistdentalgroup.com
Web: www.specialistdentalgroup.com

Specialist Dental Group is a team of experienced dental surgeons whose international qualifications include US and Canadian board certification as well as fellowships from dental governing bodies in Australia, the UK, and Singapore. Services provided include dental implants, cosmetic dentistry, teeth whitening, crowns, bridges, veneers, dentures, root canal, oral surgery, periodontal care, and orthodontics. The clinic also offers the Teeth-in-an-Hour dental implant procedure, which utilizes advanced imaging and computer design technology to enable the placement of implants and artificial replacement teeth at the same time.

Feature Story

"I Just Want to Bite an Apple!"

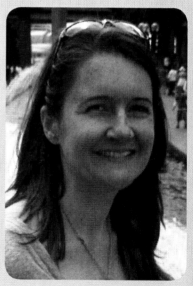

The last time she'd taken a bite out of an apple, Kristin Thompson was only 15 years old. One of her canine teeth had not developed, leaving a gap. Although a porcelain bridge had been fitted some years later to cover the two teeth on either side of the gap, biting continued to be a problem into her adulthood.

The 32-year-old freelance photographer from Columbia, Maryland, wanted to get dental implants at home, but the high cost deterred her. Then, while surfing in Indonesia in 2005, Kristin cracked the teeth holding her bridge. In excruciating pain, she made an emergency appointment with a dental surgeon who had been recommended earlier, Dr. Ansgar Cheng from the Specialist Dental Group.

An x-ray later confirmed that a large abscess in the teeth holding the bridge was causing the pain. Moreover, those chronically infected teeth were no longer strong enough to remain in place. Explaining the need to extract them, Dr. Cheng says, "A dental infection of the upper teeth may spread through blood vessels and eventually to the front part of the brain. So it was crucial to have the infection treated promptly."

Because dental implants are not usually fitted into symptomatic infected areas, Kristin first needed temporary implants. Dr. Cheng expedited the process of making them while his staff arranged her accommodation in a nearby hotel. In three days, Kristin received her temporary implants.

Although she had to go back to Singapore on several occasions over the next seven months until her permanent new teeth were fitted over the implants, Kristin has no regrets. She declares, "If I didn't know better, I'd think that these are my original teeth. The color and texture are perfectly matched, and the placement, size, and position with my gums are perfect."

"Getting dental implants changed my life for the better, but taking that first bite of an apple with them—well, the feeling is indescribable."

Surgeons International Holdings

Gleneagles Medical Centre
6 Napier Road, Suite 08-16
SINGAPORE 258499
Tel: 65 6363.3939 (24-hour hotline)
Fax: 65 6471.1088
Email: helpmail@sgih.com.sg
Web: www.sgih.com.sg

Surgeons International Holdings (SGIH) is a group of surgeons from different specialties working together to promote surgical excellence and deliver excellent patient care. Most of the surgeons in the group have been in private practice for ten to 15 years. SGIH is not confined to one hospital; as it is mobile, it can fit into any medical institution in the region and operate out of day-surgery centers.

TP Dental Surgeons

The Penthouse
391B Orchard Road
#26-01 Ngee Ann City, Tower B
SINGAPORE 238874
Tel: 65 6737.9011
Fax: 65 6732.1979
Email: contact@tpdental.com.sg
Web: www.tpdental.com.sg

Established more than 30 years ago, TP Dental Surgeons (TP Dental) is one of the largest dental surgeries practicing in a single establishment in Singapore. The TP Dental facility is housed in a 10,000-square-foot (929-square-meter) penthouse unit at the top of one of Singapore's most popular shopping centers. It has its own in-house laboratory in addition to facilities in several private hospitals for use when extensive oral surgery is required. TP Dental has 20 dental surgeons who provide the full range of general and specialty dental services to its clients, many of whom are regionally based expatriates.

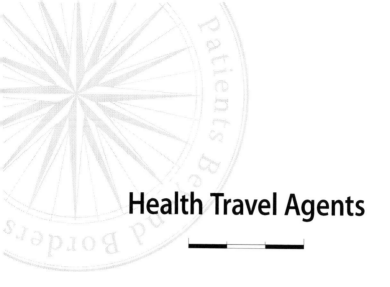

Health Travel Agents

BridgeHealth International, Inc.

5299 DTC Boulevard, Suite 800
Greenwood Village, CO 80111
Tel: 800 680.1366 (US toll-free); 303 457.5745
Fax: 303 779.0366
Email: info@bridgehealthintl.com
Web: www.bridgehealthintl.com

In 2008 BridgeHealth International (BHI) acquired Medical Tours International (MTI; see below). Together, these companies now send patients to Argentina, Brazil, China, Costa Rica, India, South Korea, Panama, Singapore, South Africa, Thailand, and Turkey. Serving the business and insurance markets as well as individual consumers, the BHI/MTI staff is composed entirely of RNs and medical care coordinators.

Before accepting a client, BHI screens for health and "travelability." Clients pay no facilitation fees; the fees are paid by BHI's approved list of physicians, clinics, and hospitals. BHI refers patients only to JCI-accredited or equivalent hospitals.

Services include passport and visa assistance, air reservations, medical consultations, medical records transfer assistance, pre-operative and post-operative counseling, followup care arrangements, and full in-country concierge services. BHI coordinates a full range of care from cosmetic, dental, bariatric, and stem cell procedures to orthopedic surgery, neurosurgery, cardiovascular surgery, and organ transplants.

Globe Health Tours

Ericht Lodge
Ashgrove Road
Blairgowrie, Perthshire, UNITED KINGDOM PH10 7BS
Tel: 203 987.5475 (US); 44 871 789.6150
Fax: 44 870 123.1672
Email: info@globehealthtours.com
Web: www.globehealthtours.com

Globe Health Tours (GHT) is a partnership between the Scottish Dental Implant Centre and HelpMeGo.To, a leading travel company in the UK. Established by medical professionals, this agency helps patients schedule treatments abroad and make the associated travel arrangements. Surgical procedures offered through GHT include cardiac, cosmetic, hip replacement, orthopedic, eye, and weight-loss surgery, as well as dental implantation. The agency's Web site provides a step-by-step instruction manual on all aspects of pre- and post-treatment, from the initial planning stage to the return home.

Healthbase Online, Inc.

287 Auburn Street
Newton, MA 02466
Tel: 888 691.4584 (US toll-free); 617 418.3436
Fax: 800 986.9230 (US toll-free)
Email: info.hb@healthbase.com
Web: www.healthbase.com

Healthbase Online is organized as a one-stop source for all medical tourism needs, connecting patients with internationally accredited hospitals in India, Thailand, Singapore, Malaysia, South Korea, Belgium, Hungary, Turkey, Mexico, Brazil, Costa Rica, the Philippines, and Panama. Healthbase is in the process of expanding its services to Taiwan, South Africa, Argentina, El Salvador, Guatemala, Poland, and the Czech Republic.

By accessing the agency's researching tool, designated "Best Website for Accessing International Medical Information for Patients/Consumers" in 2007 by Consumer Health World, registered Healthbase members can explore the various medical procedures available and the hospitals that offer them. Members are guided in their decision-making by detailed hospital reviews (including accreditation, photos, videos, maps, and more), physician profiles (qualifications, present and past appointments, and professional experience), and patient testimonials. Through this secure Web portal, members can also correspond with partner hospitals and physicians, review personalized estimates from different providers, upload and selectively share their digital medical records, and book their appointments.

Healthbase charges a flat fee for its services, which include medical and dental loan financing, travel insurance, and round-the-clock customer support. Healthbase also offers customized corporate medical tourism plans to employers and insurance companies.

International SOS

331 North Bridge Road
#17-00 Odeon Towers
SINGAPORE 188720
Tel: 65 6337.7555 (24-hour alarm center)
Email: sin.medical@internationalsos.com
Web: www.internationalsos.com

Medically supervised evacuation, such as emergency ambulance or air transportation with immigration clearance, can be arranged to and in Singapore. The world's largest provider of such a service is International SOS (ISOS), which has over 5,000 professionals operating in 70 countries.

ISOS provides medical assistance and evacuation, security services, and outsourced customer care to 82 percent of the Fortune Global 100's leading multinational corporations, insurers, and financial institutions, as well as governmental organizations.

Medical Tours International

5299 DTC Boulevard, Suite 800
Greenwood Village, CO 80111
Tel: 800 680.1366 (US toll-free); 303 457.5745
Fax: 303 779.0366
Email: info@bridgehealthintl.com
Web: www.bridgehealthintl.com

Established in 2002, Medical Tours International (MTI) initially opened its doors serving only Costa Rica. Since its recent acquisition by BridgeHealth International (BHI; see above), the agency has expanded into several other countries, including Argentina, Brazil, South Africa, and Thailand. These agencies have established relationships with a large international network of hospitals and health professionals in a variety of medical disciplines.

MTI clients pay no additional fees; the agency's fees are paid by MTI's approved physicians and clinics. MTI refers patients only to accredited clinics and board-certified physicians and surgeons. Services include booking air reservations, medical consultations, and in-country accommodations; assistance shipping medical records; and pre-operative and post-operative counseling.

Med Journeys

2020 Broadway, Suite 4C
New York, NY 10023
Tel: 888 633.5769 (US toll-free); 212 931.0557
Fax: 212 656.1134
Email: sonnyk@medjourneys.com
Web: www.medjourneys.com

This agency sends most of its clients to India, Thailand, Costa Rica, and Mexico, but it has also cemented relationships with hospitals in other countries, including Singapore, Malaysia, Turkey, and Poland. Since its establishment in 2005, Med Journeys has sent more than 350 patients abroad, and the numbers are growing.

Med Journeys' standard package includes the medical procedure, accommodations during recuperation (including three meals daily), airfare, private transportation in the host country, and premium concierge services. Extra fees are generally charged for optional tours, companions, extended stays, and added medical procedures. Med Journeys encourages clients to contact physicians directly to check references or ask questions about medical procedures. Med Journeys staff members speak Spanish, Hindi, and Thai.

MedTreks

28 West Stafford Avenue
Worthington, OH 43085
Tel: 877 269.0501 (US toll-free); 614 560.0952
Fax: 614 540.7428
Email: jlund@medtreks.com
Web: www.medtreks.com

A presence in Asia since 1949, MedTreks is intimately familiar with healthcare destinations in Singapore, Thailand, India, and Costa Rica. MedTreks has forged strong partnerships with only JCI-accredited facilities in several surgical specialties: cardiovascular, thoracic, orthopedic, gastrointestinal, and neurosurgery. It has also partnered with an international air carrier and select local hotels and serviced apartments. Consumers can obtain information on surgical costs, statistics, insurance, and benefits, as well as physician and hospital ratings, from the agency's Web site, blog, and monthly newsletter.

OliveMed Healthcare Tourism Specialist

1 Brooke Road
#02-03 Katong Plaza
SINGAPORE 429979
Tel: 65 9067.2278
Fax: 65 6346.3306
Email: enquiries@olivemed.com
Web: www.olivemed.com

OliveMed is a healthcare consultancy firm linking overseas patients to various healthcare options in Singapore. It provides a full range of services from pre-departure medical consultation, medical appointment scheduling, and customized travel itinerary to post-arrival personal butler service, transportation, and concierge services.

In addition to comprehensive information about Singapore's attractions and medical services, OliveMed's Web site presents a series of videos featuring disease introduction and education by selected specialists. OliveMed has also put a bit of fun into the business by launching the world's first medical travel game, in which winners receive free health screening trips to Singapore.

Overseas Medical Services, Canada, Inc.

1771 First Avenue NW
Calgary, Alberta, CANADA T2N 0B2
Tel: 866 449.4947 (US and Canada toll-free); 403 283.4947
Fax: 403 283.2368
Email: overseasmedicalservices@gmail.com
Web: www.overseasmedicalservices.com

A pioneer of medical tourism in Canada, Overseas Medical Services, Canada, Inc. (OMS) also has affiliate offices in Florida, Oregon, and Hawaii. This agency sends patients overseas for a range of procedures that includes cosmetic surgery, oncology, dental surgery, vascular and brain surgery, joint replacements, and other orthopedic surgeries. Additional services include travel and visa arrangement for US and Canadian citizens, financing, and off-shore insurance. OMS ensures that all of its approved medical facilities provide airport transfers, interpreter services, and wheelchair-accessible accommodations at negotiated fees. OMS has recently partnered with ParkwayHealth to serve medical travelers to Singapore.

Planet Hospital

23679 Calabasas Road, Suite 150
Calabasas, CA 91302
Tel: 800 243.0172 (US toll-free); 818 665.4801
Fax: 818 665.4810
Email: rudy@planethospital.com
Web: www.planethospital.com

Rudy Rupak founded Planet Hospital in 2002, after being impressed with the quality of care his fiancée received when she fell ill in Thailand. This agency has since sent more than 1,200 patients abroad for medical care. Planet Hospital currently serves 13 countries: India, Belgium, Costa Rica, Mexico, Singapore, Thailand, South Korea, Malaysia, the Philippines, Panama, El Salvador, Cyprus, and Malta. The company has concierges in every city it serves, to take care of clients from the moment they land to the moment they leave. Planet Hospital representatives personally inspect every hospital and doctor the company recommends.

Planet Hospital currently serves several self-insured employers who have contracted with the agency to help their employees save money. Specialties include cardiovascular services, orthopedics, cosmetic surgery, dental care, fertility/reproduction (including surrogacy), and oncology. Planet Hospital is the only medical travel agency that has been a member of the Better Business Bureau since 2002 with an AA rating.

The company's Web site offers a comprehensive list of major hospitals in its service areas, along with a sampling of its top recommended physicians and their credentials. A robust testimonials page features real clients with real names. At this writing, Planet Hospital is sending five patients per day abroad for treatment from its offices in California, Saudi Arabia, the UK, Canada, and France.

The Taj Medical Group, Limited

The TechnoCentre, Coventry University Technology Park
Puma Way
Coventry, UNITED KINGDOM CV1 2TT
Tel: 877 799.9797 (US toll-free); 44 2476 466.118
Fax: 44 2476 466.118
Email: info@tajmedical.com
Web: www.tajmedical.com

and

The Taj Medical Group
408 West 57th Street, Suite 9N
New York, NY 10019
Tel: 877 799.9797 (US toll-free)
Email: info@tajmedical.com
Web: www.tajmedical.com

and

The Taj Medical Group
9513 Brant Lane
Glen Allen, VA 23060
Tel: 877 799.9797 (US toll-free)
Email: info@tajmedical.com
Web: www.tajmedical.com

Based in the UK with offices in India, Singapore, the US, and Canada, Taj Medical Group cofounders Jag and Dipa Jethwa have sent more than 1,000 patients to India over the past four years, mostly from Canada, Great Britain, and parts of Europe. Taj's new US offices in New York City and Virginia were opened in 2007 to facilitate the needs of American health travelers.

Taj has longstanding formal partnerships with many hospitals in India, including Escorts Heart Institute, Apollo Hospitals Group, Wockhardt Hospitals, and Max Healthcare. Taj has recently expanded its hospital partnerships and now sends clients to JCI-accredited hospitals in the UK, Germany, Singapore, Malaysia, South Korea, Thailand, and South America as well. Taj uses its extensive physician contacts to match each patient's requirements with the best physician, procedure, provider, and price.

All Taj staffers speak fluent English, and Taj insists that all their recommended physicians and surgeons be highly experienced and internationally qualified (often UK-trained or US board-certified). All the doctors speak English, too. Taj charges no upfront fees, and the agency provides all pre-travel planning, pre-operative consultation, and post-operative consultation and checkups, along with full, personal, in-country concierge service.

World Choice Healthcare

Tel: 866 631.5556 (US toll-free)
Web: www.worldchoicehealthcare.com

World Choice Healthcare (WCH) facilitates medical travel to Costa Rica, India, Malaysia, Singapore, and Thailand. Specialties offered include cosmetic, dental, orthopedic, cardiology, and selected general surgery procedures. The WCH Web site offers comprehensive information on each destination, including images of the agency's partner healthcare institutions, and features reports from its patients on the "News and Testimonials" page. WCH has affiliated with ParkwayHealth in Singapore.

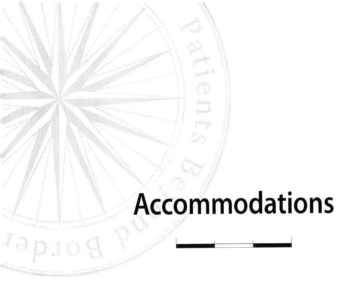

Accommodations

Singapore offers a wide variety of accommodation types to suit all budgets and preferences. They range from backpacker, budget, and youth hostels to boutique and five-star hotels. Most hotels come with standard facilities and amenities, such as international direct dial (IDD) phones, Internet and cable, room service, mini-bars, dataports for modems, nonsmoking rooms or floors, and business and fitness centers furnished with the latest equipment.

Different accommodation types are situated across most parts of Singapore; therefore, it is easy to find a suitable accommodation close to any medical facility.

Useful Information

Rates and Reservations

You are strongly advised to make advance reservations to avoid disappointment. Most major credit cards are accepted; you may be required to leave a credit card imprint or number upon checking in. Rates are usually quoted in Singapore dollars and may be subject to a 10 percent service charge, as well as a 7 percent Goods and Services Tax (GST).

Getting to Your Hotel

You can reach every corner of the island with Singapore's modern, efficient, and reliable public transportation system, which consists of a bus network and a mass rapid transit (MRT) rail system. Taxis are numerous and affordable. Detailed information on bus routes, MRT stations, and fares can be found in the *TransitLink Guide,* which can be purchased at bus interchanges, MRT stations, and major bookstores in Singapore; alternatively, this information is also available at www.sbstransit.com.sg.

Hotel Phone Services

Most hotels offer in-room IDD telephone services. Some hotels may charge a minimum 30-cent surcharge. Generally, local calls are charged at 10 Singapore cents for every three minutes.

Accommodations Listing

Name	Details	Type
Albert Court Hotel	180 Albert Street Singapore 189971 Tel: 65 6339.3939 Fax: 65 6339.3253 Email: info@albertcourt.com.sg Web: www.albertcourt.com.sg	Hotel (moderate)

Name	Details	Type
Allson Hotel Singapore	101 Victoria Street Singapore 188018 Tel: 65 6336.0811 Fax: 65 6339.0631 Email: allson.res@pacific.net.sg Web: www.allsonhotelsingapore.com	Hotel (moderate)
Carlton Hotel Singapore	76 Bras Basah Road Singapore 189558 Tel: 65 6338.8333 Fax: 65 6339.6866 Email: mail@carltonhotel.sg Web: www.carlton.com.sg	Hotel (deluxe)
Changi Hotel Singapore	80 Changi Road Singapore 419715 Tel: 65 6346.3388 Fax: 65 6345.7661 Email: changihotel@pacific.net.sg Web: www.oxfordhotel.com.sg/ changi/index.htm	Hotel (moderate)
Conrad Centennial Singapore	2 Temasek Boulevard Singapore 038982 Tel: 65 6334.8888 Fax: 65 6333.9166 Email: singaporeinfo@conradhotels.com Web: singapore.conradmeetings.com	Hotel (deluxe)
Copthorne King's Hotel	403 Havelock Road Singapore 169632 Tel: 65 6733.0011 Fax: 65 6732.5764 Email: rooms@copthornekings.com.sg Web: www.copthornekings.com.sg	Hotel (moderate)
Copthorne Orchid Hotel Singapore	214 Dunearn Road Singapore 299526 Tel: 65 6415.6000 Fax: 65 6250.9292 Email: rsvn@copthorneorchid.com.sg Web: www.copthorneorchid.com.sg	Hotel (deluxe)
The Elizabeth Hotel	24 Mount Elizabeth Singapore 228518 Tel: 65 6738.1188 Fax: 65 6732.3866 Email: pr@theelizabeth.com.sg Web: www.theelizabeth.com.sg	Hotel (deluxe)

Name	Details	Type
Fairmont Singapore	80 Bras Basah Road Singapore 189560 Tel: 65 6339.7777 Fax: 65 6338.1554 Email: singapore@fairmont.com Web: www.fairmont.com/singapore	Hotel (deluxe)
Far East Plaza Residences	14 Scotts Road Singapore 228213 Tel: 65 6428.8600 Fax: 65 6438.7128 Email: lease-svc@fareast.com.sg Web: www.fareastsvcapts.com.sg/ fe-intro.asp	Serviced Apartments
Four Seasons Hotel Singapore	190 Orchard Boulevard Singapore 248646 Tel: 65 6831.7305 Fax: 65 6733.0669 Web: www.fourseasons.com/singapore	Hotel (deluxe)
Fraser Suites River Valley Singapore	491A River Valley Road Singapore 248372 Tel: 65 6737.5800 Fax: 65 6737.5560 Email: sales.singapore@frasershospitality .com Web: singapore-suites.frasershospitality .com	Serviced Apartments
Furama Riverfront Singapore	405 Havelock Road Singapore 169633 Tel: 65 6333.8898 Fax: 65 6733.1588 Email: riverfront@furama.com Web: www.furama.com/riverfront	Hotel (deluxe)
Golden Landmark Hotel, Singapore	390 Victoria Street Singapore 188061 Tel: 65 6297.2828 Fax: 65 6298.2038 Email: info@goldenlandmark.com.sg Web: www.goldenlandmark.com.sg	Hotel (moderate)
Goodwood Park Singapore	22 Scotts Road Singapore 228221 Tel: 65 6737.7411 Fax: 65 6732.8558 Email: enquiries@goodwoodpark hotel.com Web: www.goodwoodparkhotel.com	Hotel (deluxe)

Name	Details	Type
Grand Copthorne Singapore Waterfront Hotel	392 Havelock Road Singapore 169663 Tel: 65 6733.0880 Fax: 65 6737.8880 Email: frontoffice@grandcopthorne.com.sg Web: www.grandcopthorne.com.sg	Hotel (deluxe)
Grand Hyatt Singapore	10 Scotts Road Singapore 228211 Tel: 65 6738.1234 Fax: 65 6732.1696 Email: singapore.grand@hyatt.com Web: www.singapore.grand.hyatt.com	Hotel (deluxe)
Grand Mercure Roxy Hotel	50 East Coast Road Roxy Square Singapore 428769 Tel: 65 6344.8000 (hotel code 3610) Fax: 65 6344.8010 Email: info@grandmercureroxy.com.sg Web: www.mercure.com/mercure/fichehotel/gb/mer/3610/fiche_hotel.shtml	Hotel (moderate)
Hangout @ Mt. Emily	10A Upper Wilkie Road Singapore 228119 Tel: 65 6438.5588 Fax: 65 6339.6008 Email: enquiries@hangouthotels.com Web: www.hangouthotels.com	Hotel (boutique)
Hilton Singapore	581 Orchard Road Singapore 238883 Tel: 65 6737.2233 Fax: 65 6732.2917 Email: singapore@hilton.com Web: www.singapore.hilton.com	Hotel (deluxe)
Holiday Inn Atrium Singapore	317 Outram Road Singapore 169075 Tel: 65 6733.0188 Fax: 65 6733.0989 Email: hiatrium@hiatrium.com Web: www.holiday-inn.com/atrium-sin	Hotel (deluxe)
Holiday Inn Park View Singapore	11 Cavenagh Road Singapore 229616 Tel: 65 6733.8333 Fax: 65 6734.4593 Email: info@hiparkview.com Web: www.holiday-inn.com/sin-parkview	Hotel (deluxe)

Name	Details	Type
Hotel Miramar	401 Havelock Road Singapore 169631 Tel: 65 6733.0222 Fax: 65 6733.4027 Email: miramar@pacific.net.sg Web: www.miramar.com.sg	Hotel (moderate)
Hotel Royal	36 Newton Road Singapore 307964 Tel: 65 6426.0168 Fax: 65 6253.8668 Email: royal@hotelroyal.com.sg Web: www.hotelroyal.com.sg	Hotel (moderate)
Intercontinental Singapore	80 Middle Road Singapore 188966 Tel: 65 6338.7600 Fax: 65 6338.7366 Email: singapore@interconti.com Web: www.singapore.intercontinental.com	Hotel (deluxe)
Lanson Place Winsland Serviced Residences	167 Penang Road Singapore 238462 Tel: 65 6833.0704 Fax: 65 6833.0705 Email: enquiry.lpws@lansonplace.com Web: www.lansonplace.com/lansonSG.html	Serviced Apartments
Link Hotel	50 Tiong Bahru Road Singapore 168733 Tel: 65 6622.8585 Fax: 65 6622.8558 Email: info@linkhotel.com.sg Web: www.linkhotel.com.sg	Hotel (boutique)
Meritus Mandarin Singapore	333 Orchard Road Singapore 238867 Tel: 65 6737.4411 Fax: 65 6732.2361 Email: mandarin.tms@meritus-hotels.com Web: www.mandarin-singapore.com	Hotel (deluxe)
Naumi Hotel	41 Seah Street Singapore 188396 Tel: 65 6403.6000 Fax: 65 6403.6010 Email: naumiaide@naumihotel.com Web: www.naumihotel.com	Hotel (boutique)

Name	Details	Type
New Majestic Hotel	31-37 Bukit Pasoh Road Singapore 089845 Tel: 65 6511.4700 Fax: 65 6347.1923 Email: reservation@newmajestichotel .com Web: www.newmajestichotel.com	Hotel (boutique)
New Orchid Hotel	347 Balestier Road Singapore 329777 Tel: 65 6253.2112 Fax: 65 6255.6033 Email: neworchidhotel@hotmail.com Web: www.avipclub.com/sg/neworchid	Hotel (moderate)
Orchard Hotel Singapore	442 Orchard Road Singapore 238879 Tel: 65 6734.7766 Fax: 65 6733.5482 Email: enquiry@orchardhotel.com.sg Web: www.orchardhotel.com.sg	Hotel (deluxe)
Orchard Parade Hotel	1 Tanglin Road Singapore 247905 Tel: 65 6737.1133 Fax: 65 6733.0242 Email: info@orchardparade.com.sg Web: www.orchardparade.com.sg	Hotel (deluxe)
Orchard Scotts Residences	5 Anthony Road Singapore 229954 Tel: 65 6428.8688 Fax: 65 6438.7128 Email: enquiry@orchardscotts.com.sg Web: www.orchardscotts.com.sg	Serviced Apartments
Pan Pacific Orchard	10 Claymore Road Singapore 229540 Tel: 65 6831.6682 Fax: 65 737.9075 Email: orchard@panpacific.com Web: www.panpacific.com/orchard	Hotel (deluxe)
Paramount Hotel	25 Marine Parade Singapore 449536 Tel: 65 6344.2200 Fax: 65 6447.4131 Email: par.reservation@ytchotels.com.sg Web: www.ytchotels.com.sg/sp-ytcparam	Hotel (moderate)

Name	Details	Type
Park Hotel Orchard	270 Orchard Road Singapore 238857 Tel: 65 6732.1111 Fax: 65 6732.7018 Email: info@orsg.parkhotelgroup.com Web: www.parkhotelgroup.com/phorch/ phorchoo_index.html	Hotel (deluxe)
Parkroyal on Beach Road, Singapore	7500 Beach Road Singapore 199591 Tel: 65 6298.0011 Fax: 65 6296.3600 Email: enquiry@br.parkroyalhotels.sg Web: www.beach.singapore.parkroyal hotels.com	Hotel (deluxe)
Parkroyal Residences	7500A Beach Road #01-345/346 The Plaza Singapore 199591 Tel: 65 6296.2511 Fax: 65 6293.8158 Email: apartment@hpl.com.sg Web: www.uol.com.sg/pr	Serviced Apartments
Park View Hotel	81 Beach Road Singapore 189692 Tel: 65 6338.8558 Fax: 65 6334.8558 Email: parkview@parkview.com.sg Web: www.parkview.com.sg	Hotel (moderate)
Quality Hotel Singapore	201 Balestier Road Singapore 329926 Tel: 65 6355.9988 Fax: 65 6255.0998 Email: reservation@qualityhotel.com.sg Web: www.qualityhotel.com.sg	Hotel (moderate)
Raffles Hotel	1 Beach Road Singapore 189673 Tel: 65 6337.1886 Fax: 65 6339.7650 Email: singapore@raffles.com Web: www.raffleshotel.com	Hotel (deluxe)
The Regent Singapore	1 Cuscaden Road Singapore 249715 Tel: 65 6733.8888 Fax: 65 6738.8838 Email: reservation.rsn@fourseasons.com Web: www.regenthotels.com/singapore	Hotel (deluxe)

Name	Details	Type
The Ritz-Carlton, Millenia Singapore	7 Raffles Avenue Singapore 039799 Tel: 65 6337.8888 Fax: 65 6338.0001 Web: www.ritzcarlton.com/en/ properties/singapore	Hotel (deluxe)
River View Hotel Singapore	382 Havelock Road Singapore 169629 Tel: 65 6732.9922 Fax: 65 6732.1034 Email: reservation@riverview.com.sg Web: www.riverview.com.sg	Hotel (deluxe)
Royal Plaza on Scotts	25 Scotts Road Singapore 228220 Tel: 65 6737.7966 Fax: 65 6737.6646 Email: royal@royalplaza.com.sg Web: www.royalplaza.com.sg	Hotel (deluxe)
The Scarlet Hotel	33 Erskine Road Singapore 069333 Tel: 65 6511.3333 Fax: 65 6511.3303 Email: reservations@thescarlethotel.com Web: www.thescarlethotel.com	Hotel (boutique)
Shangri-La Hotel Singapore	22 Orange Grove Road Singapore 258350 Tel: 65 6737.3644 Fax: 65 6737.3257 Email: sls@shangri-la.com Web: www.shangri-la.com/en/property/ singapore/shangrila	Hotel (deluxe)
Sheraton Towers Singapore	39 Scotts Road Singapore 228230 Tel: 65 6737.6888 Fax: 65 6737.1072 Email: sheraton.towers.singapore@ sheraton.com Web: www.sheratonsingapore.com	Hotel (deluxe)
Singapore Marriott Hotel	320 Orchard Road Singapore 238865 Tel: 65 6735.5800 Fax: 65 6735.9800 Email: mhrs.sindt.sales@marriotthotels.com Web: www.singaporemarriott.com	Hotel (deluxe)

Name	Details	Type
Somerset Bencoolen Residences	51 Bencoolen Street Singapore 189630 Tel: 65 6849.4688 Fax: 65 6849.4700 Email: enquiry.singapore@the-ascott.com Web: www.somersetbencoolen.com	Serviced Apartments
Somerset Compass	2 Mount Elizabeth Link Singapore 227973 Tel: 65 6732.7737 Fax: 65 6732.8068 Email: enquiry.singapore@the-ascott.com Web: www.somersetcompass.com	Serviced Apartments
Swissotel Merchant Court Singapore	20 Merchant Court Singapore 058281 Tel: 65 6337.2288 Fax: 65 6334.0606 Email: singapore-merchantcourt@swissotel.com Web: www.swissotel.com/singapore-merchantcourt	Hotel (deluxe)
Swissotel The Stamford Singapore	2 Stamford Road Singapore 178882 Tel: 65 6338.8585 Fax: 65 6338.2862 Email: emailus.singapore@swissotel.com Web: www.swissotel-thestamford.com	Hotel (deluxe)
Traders Hotel Singapore	1A Cuscaden Road Singapore 249716 Tel: 65 6738.2222 Fax: 65 6831.4314 Email: ths@shangri-la.com Web: www.shangri-la.com/en/property/singapore/traders	Hotel (deluxe)
Treetops Executive Residences	7 Orange Grove Road Singapore 258355 Tel: 65 6887.0088 Fax: 65 6887.0066 Email: sales@treetops.com.sg Web: www.treetops.com.sg	Serviced Apartments
York Hotel Singapore	21 Mount Elizabeth Singapore 228516 Tel: 65 6737.0511 Fax: 65 6732.1217 Email: enquiry@yorkhotel.com.sg Web: www.yorkhotel.com.sg	Hotel (deluxe)

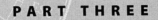

PART THREE

Uniquely Singapore

Singapore in a Nutshell

Early History

The history of Singapore begins with an intriguing blend of fact and myth in the second century. The earliest written record of Singapore is a third-century Chinese account describing it as *Pu-luo-chung* or "island at the tip of a peninsula." By 1365 the island had become part of the mighty Sri Vijayan Empire and was known as *Temasek*, which is the Javanese word for "sea town." Legend holds that in the fourteenth century, a visiting Sri Vijayan prince, Sang Nila Utama, saw an animal he mistook for a lion — and thus Singapore's modern name of *Singa Pura* or "lion city" was born.

Singapore is among the 20 smallest countries in the world, with a total land area of only 272 square miles (704 square kilometers). The US is about 15,000 times bigger.

The British wrote the next notable chapter in Singapore's history. In 1819 an official of the British East India Company, Sir Stamford Raffles, combed the Straits of Malacca looking for a small trading station to counter the Dutch influence in the area — and the tiny fishing village of Singapore, at the crossroads of the East and the West, was perfect. When Sir Raffles then proclaimed the island a free port, this policy of free trade attracted merchants from all over Asia and from as far away as the US and the Middle East.

As a British colony, in 1832 Singapore became the center of government for its fellow Straits Settlements of Penang and Malacca. The opening of the Suez Canal in 1869 and the advent of telegraph and steamship increased Singapore's importance as a hub for expanding trade between East and West.

> Singapore has more than 1,864 miles (3,000 kilometers) of roads. Stretched end to end, they would reach all the way from Singapore to Hong Kong.

Singapore had been the site of military action in the fourteenth century, when it became embroiled in the struggle for the Malay Peninsula between Siam (now Thailand) and the Java-based Majapahit Empire. Five centuries later, it was again the scene of significant fighting during World War II. Singapore was considered an impregnable fortress, but Japanese forces overran the island in 1942. After the war, Singapore again became a Crown Colony. The growth of nationalism led to self-government in 1959, and on August 9, 1965, Singapore became an independent republic.

Heritage and Geography

Singapore has retained its special multiracial quality since the early days when Arabs, Chinese, Europeans, Indians, and Straits-born Chinese (or Peranakans) came to live side by side with the indigenous Malays. Today the country's three main ethnic groups (Chinese, Malays, and Indians) as well as Eurasians complement and supplement each other, while each group retains its individual cultural identity.

Situated at one of the crossroads of the world, Singapore occupies a strategic location that has boosted its growth into a major international center for trade, communications, and tourism. The island is about 85 miles (137 kilometers) north of the equator, between latitudes 1030°38' east and 1040°06' east. It is linked to Malaysia by two causeway bridges, and the major islands of Indonesia's Riau Archipelago are a quick ferry ride away. Thailand and the Philippines are within a short journey by plane.

> Despite being largely urbanized, Singapore is the largest exporter of ornamental fish, with 25 percent of the world market.

Singapore's National Symbol: The Merlion

First designed as an emblem for Singapore in 1964, the merlion resting on a crest of waves quickly became the country's icon to the rest of the world. The merlion's leonine head represents the legendary beast spotted by Prince Sang Nila Utama, and its fish tail symbolizes ancient Temasek, representing Singapore's humble beginnings as a fishing village.

Singapore Is Unique

If there is one word that best captures Singapore, that word is *unique*. A dynamic city rich in contrast and color, Singapore is a harmonious blend of cultures, cuisines, arts, and architectural styles, brimming with unbridled energy. This little dynamo in Southeast Asia embodies the finest of both East and West, offering the modern and cosmopolitan while at the same time retaining its distinctive local flavor. A single day's walking tour can take you from the past to the future, from exotic ethnic enclaves to efficient business centers, and from serene gardens to sleek skyscrapers.

For more information about Singapore's history, attractions, and accommodations, visit the Uniquely Singapore site, www.visit singapore.com.

Twenty Unique Things to Do in Singapore

1. Be serenaded at Jurong Bird Park

Jurong Bird Park is the largest bird park in Southeast Asia. Attractions include the Waterfall Aviary, the world's highest artificial waterfall at nearly 100 feet (30 meters); the Penguin Parade, where penguins live and play in an environment similar to that of the South Pole; and the Southeast Asia Birds Aviary, where a thunderstorm is simulated every day at noon. Take flight only after enjoying refreshments at the Lodge on Flamingo Lake, overlooking the tastefully landscaped home of more than a thousand flamingoes. For more information, see www.birdpark .com.sg.

2. Tour the city on a DUCK

The fun begins once you board the Duck, an amphibious, American military craft once used in the Vietnam War. The friendly

DUCKtour crew guides you on an hour-long city and heritage trail on both land and water — probably the most unusual mode of sightseeing around Singapore. For more information, see www.ducktours.com.sg.

3. Rediscover the wonders of science at the Science Centre Singapore

This themed attraction is fun for the whole family, with a range of interesting and interactive exhibits. Explore the Kinetic Garden, Asia's first outdoor interactive science garden. The specially designed Omni-Theatre next door, equipped with state-of-the-art IMAX dome technology, contains a massive hemispheric screen that displays the largest film-size format in the history of motion pictures. For more information, see www.science.edu.sg.

The Bukit Timah Nature Reserve in Singapore contains more species of trees than are found on the entire North American continent.

4. Catch a glimpse of Singapore's colonial roots at Raffles Hotel

Restored to its 1920s grandeur, this grand old dame is world renowned for its charm and elegance. Singapore's oldest hotel has played host to famous celebrities and writers, such as Somerset Maugham and Joseph Conrad. Sip a refreshing Singapore Sling at the Long Bar, the birthplace of this popular cocktail. For more information, see www.raffleshotel.com.

5. Melt your cares away at Spa Botanica

Nestled in beautiful greenery on the hillside of Sentosa Island, Singapore's first garden spa is a haven devoted to the art of rejuvenation. Spa Botanica blends indoor pampering with outdoor treatments to draw on the healing powers of nature. For more information, see www.spabotanica.com.

6. Immerse yourself in the arts at the Esplanade–Theatres on the Bay

Many of Singapore's performing arts venues and institutions are more than just performance locations — they are architectural marvels in their own right. Lovingly dubbed "the Durians" by locals for its roofs resembling that prickly tropical fruit, the Esplanade–Theatres on the Bay is Singapore's most exciting performing arts complex to date. Catch an evening concert or drama at the Esplanade's 1,600-seat concert hall, 2,000-seat theater, recital rooms, or outdoor performance spaces. For more information, see www.esplanade.com.

> The Singapore Sling was first served in 1915 at the Long Bar of the Raffles Hotel.

7. Shop for unique souvenirs in Singapore's ethnic districts

The ethnic quarters around the city's center brim with local foodstuffs and cultural items, as well as arts and antiques from all over the world that make wonderful gifts. From traditional

Chinese medicine in Chinatown and beautiful fabrics on Arab Street in Kampong Glam, to beaded Peranakan slippers in Katong and saris and spices in Little India, there are treasures aplenty to be discovered.

8. "Sky Dine" on a cable car

Escape from the city for an amazing dining experience at 200 feet (more than 70 meters) above the sea aboard a cable car. You will savor delicious continental delights while enjoying the panoramic evening skyline of the city and harbor. For more information, see www.mountfaber.com.sg/main-skydining.htm.

9. Take a ferry to Bintan Resorts

Less than an hour from Singapore via a comfortable ferry ride, Bintan Resorts are located on the largest of Indonesia's Riau Islands in the South China Sea. Experience Bintan's endless beaches, a wide variety of international-class resorts, and a refreshing host of tropical holiday activities. For more information, see www.bintan-resorts.com.

10. Play an old game with a new twist

What better way to take home a slice of Singapore than to buy up local properties — Monopoly style? The Uniquely Singapore (Special Edition) Monopoly set features Singapore landmarks and locations for sale, as well as new game-pieces in the form of Singapore icons, such as the trishaw and the Kucinta cat.

11. "Chill out" at Boat Quay

Boat Quay was once the busiest part of the old Port of Singapore, handling three-quarters of all shipping business during the 1860s. The nineteenth-century shops along the river now house various bars, pubs, and restaurants, set against a stunning backdrop of modern skyscrapers — a perfect stage for a casual night out.

12. Honor World War II heroes and memories at Changi Chapel and Museum

Built by Changi Prison inmates, the Changi Chapel and Museum stands as a monument to those who maintained their faith and dignity during those dark years. Letters, photographs, drawings, and personal effects in the museum relate the agony of the Japanese Occupation and the imprisonment of more than 50,000 civilians and soldiers in Singapore. For more information, see www.changimuseum.com.

13. See animals in a different light at the Night Safari

The world's first zoo designed for visiting at night, the Night Safari uses subtle lighting techniques to offer the experience of viewing more than 1,000 nocturnal animals of 100 species in their vast natural habitats. At the interactive "Creatures of the Night" show, visitors can get up close and personal with owls, bats, otters, a giant python, and more. For more information, see www.nightsafari.com.sg.

14. Uncover layers of history along the Singapore River

Stroll along the Singapore River and you will encounter a series of lifelike, life-sized bronze sculptures. Called the "People of the River," these sculptures depict the lifestyles of the riverside's early inhabitants, creating an arresting picture of Singapore's growth from a small river settlement to a bustling city.

15. Get your feet tickled at Fish Reflexology

Experience a unique and revitalizing therapy at Fish Reflexology in Underwater World, Sentosa. Relax your feet in a warm pool, and soon a school of Turkish spa fish will swim up and gently nibble at your toes. These little fish consume only dead skin areas — a perfect and most unusual way to exfoliate and pamper your feet. For more information, see www.underwaterworld.com.sg/fishreflex.htm.

> Singapore's Night Safari is the world's first "night zoo."

16. Trace the growth of Tiger Beer at TigerLIVE

TigerLIVE is a multimedia, multisensory entertainment center that takes visitors through the growth of Singapore's renowned Tiger Beer, from its beginnings in the 1930s to its emergence in modern times as a world-acclaimed brand and winner of numerous international awards. Enjoy a fresh brew while you are there. For more information, see www.tigerlive.com.sg.

17. Savor fresh seafood by the East Coast beach

Away from the city, the East Coast is the quintessential beachfront relaxation spot for travelers. Taste Singapore's signature chili crab, black pepper crab, and other sumptuous dishes at the East Coast Seafood Centre, where several major seafood restaurants vie for your palate.

The 2008 Formula 1 SingTel Singapore Grand Prix in September 2008 was not only F1's first street race in Asia but also the first-ever night race in F1 history.

18. Take in a complete overview of Singapore on the Singapore Flyer

The world's largest observation wheel, the Singapore Flyer stands at 541 feet (165 meters)—about 98 feet (30 meters) taller than the famed London Eye. A flight on this SGD240 million wheel offers you a 360° visual feast of Singapore and beyond. For more information, see www.singaporeflyer.com.

19. Shop 'til you drop at Mustafa Centre

Open around the clock, this six-story shopping center is a treasure trove of discount shopping, carrying everything from skincare products and diamonds to electronics and sportswear. Customers claim that merchandise at Mustafa

The largest fountain in the world is located at Suntec City in Singapore. Made of cast bronze, it cost US$6 million to build in 1997.

Centre is much cheaper than elsewhere. For more information, see www.mustafa.com.sg.

20. Imagine life in one of Singapore's public housing estates

Visit Tampines (pronounced "Tam-pe-nees"), a public housing estate in the eastern part of Singapore that has won the coveted United Nations World Habitat Award for Excellent Housing Design. It boasts all the facilities that residents could want, including schools, markets, shops, playgrounds, and a sports stadium.

Dietary Cautions for Medical Travelers

The fabulous foods of Singapore will tempt you at every turn, but in the days before or after a surgical or medical procedure, it is wise to limit your culinary experimentation. Your stomach may not be ready for new taste sensations, especially if you are taking medication. Plan to delight in Singapore's abundant cuisines when you are completely well—and always follow your doctor's dietary instructions to the letter.

PART FOUR

Resources
and References

ADDITIONAL RESOURCES

Other Editions of Patients Beyond Borders

Each year Healthy Travel Media publishes new, specialized editions of *Patients Beyond Borders*. Country-specific editions include Singapore, Korea, Taiwan, India, and Malaysia. A treatment-specific series is coming soon as well, beginning with *Patients Beyond Borders: Orthopedic Edition*. Visit www.patientsbeyondborders.com to check on special editions for your destination or treatment.

World, Country, and City Information

The World Factbook. Cataloged by country, *The World Factbook* — compiled by the US Central Intelligence Agency (CIA) — is an excellent source of general, up-to-date information about the geography, economy, and history of countries around the world. Go to www.cia.gov; in the left column, find "Library and Reference," then click on "The World Factbook."

Lonely Planet. This feisty travel book publisher has compiled a collection of useful online snippets (mostly as teasers to get you to buy the books) along with useful links. Go to www.lonelyplanet.com and search for your country of interest to find information on transport, events, and more.

Becoming Informed Here and Abroad

You: The Smart Patient: An Insider's Guide for Getting the Best Treatment. Physicians Michael F. Roizen and Mehmet C. Oz have written a witty, often irreverent, and highly useful guide to becoming an informed patient, whether in your doctor's office or dentist's chair, on the surgeon's table, or in an emergency room. This 400-page consumer bible is packed with information on patients' rights, surgical precautions, second and third opinions, health insurance plans, health records, and precautionary advice that falls outside the scope of this book.

World Travel Guide. The publishers of the *Columbus World Travel Guide* sponsor the Web site www.worldtravelguide .net, which offers good information on countries and major metropolitan areas throughout the world. Go to the site's "Choose Guide" search to find information on airports, tours, attractions, cruises, and more.

Singapore Sources

SingaporeMedicine. More than 400,000 international patients go to Singapore each year for medical care ranging from health screening to heart and brain surgeries. Whether their needs are simple or complex, patients find assurance in a world-class healthcare system that emphasizes safety and excellence. Learn more at www.singaporemedicine.com.

Visiting Singapore. Discover the many attractions and events that delight international travelers to Singapore. Check out www.visitsingapore.com for information on what to eat, what to see, and what to do during your visit. There's a currency converter on the Web site, too.

World Atlas

Google Earth. If you've not downloaded Google Earth, go there and do so. It's truly one of the wonders of the online world. After you download it, you can zoom to your home's rooftop or "fly" to any continent, country, or city on the planet simply by typing in the appropriate keywords. Legends include city names, roads, terrain, populated places, borders, 3-D buildings, and more. Go to http:// earth.google.com/ and follow the download instructions.

Encarta Atlas. Encarta, Microsoft's easy-to-use, free atlas, allows you to quickly click your way around the planet and then obtain information on your country of interest. Go to www.encarta.com and click on the "World Atlas" tab.

Passports and Visas

Travisa. Dozens of online agencies offer visa services. We've found Travisa, at www.travisa.com, to be reliable and accessible by telephone as well. The agency offers good customer service and followup. Travisa's Web site also carries links to information on immunization requirements, travel warnings, current weather, and more.

Currency Converter

www.xe.com. To learn quickly how much your money is worth in your country of interest, go to www.xe.com and click on "Quick Currency Converter."

Traveler's Tips

Smart Packing by Susan Foster (Third Edition, Smart Travel Press, 2008) includes timely information on airport security, airline regulations, and travel security. It offers advice on luggage selection, matching clothes to the occasion, and finding the right fabrics and styles for every season. The book also includes chapters on how to travel light and what to do about toiletries, cosmetics, electrical appliances, and travel gadgets.

International Hospital Accreditation

Joint Commission International. Mentioned frequently throughout this book, the Joint Commission International (JCI) remains the only game in town for international hospital accreditation. To see a current list of accredited hospitals by country, go to www.jointcommission international.org.

Medical Dictionary

Merriam-Webster's Medical Dictionary. If a multisyllabic medical term stumps you, don't run out and purchase an unabridged brick of a medical dictionary. Several free, online medical glossaries offer more than you probably want to know on most health topics. *Merriam-Webster's Medical Dictionary* is provided on a number of sites, including MedlinePlus (http://medlineplus.gov) and InteliHealth (www.intelihealth.com). The simplest access is through http://dictionary.reference.com. Just type in a medical word or phrase and voila! For a richer exploration of a given medical term, MedicineNet (www.medicinenet.com) and similar sources offer articles, services, and a thicket of sponsored links.

Medical Information

MedlinePlus is a US government-sponsored medical site that brings together a wealth of information from the National Library of Medicine (the world's largest medical library), the National Institutes of Health, *Merriam-Webster's Medical Dictionary,* the *United States Pharmacopeia,* and other sources. Go to http://medlineplus.gov and click any of the various choices in the left column. The online tour at www.nlm.nih.gov/medlineplus/tour/medlineplustour.html helps you navigate this massive site.

Medical Travel Resources

Medical Tourism Insight is a monthly online newsletter written for the medical travel industry as well as employers, benefits managers, government officials, and prospective patients. Coverage includes objective and timely information on overseas medical care and related issues, such as health insurance and employee health benefits. The Web site is www.medical tourisminsight.com.

The *International Medical Travel Journal (IMTJ)* is a prominent online journal for the medical travel industry. While geared more toward industry professionals than consumers, it does provide a free online guide for potential patients at www.imtjonline.com. There's a free email newsletter, too, and a paid subscription service for those who are serious about industry news.

International Society of Travel Medicine. If you are looking for information about immunizations, infectious diseases, or other aspects of medical travel, check out the Web site of the International Society of Travel Medicine (ISTM) at www.istm.org. This organization maintains offices in Georgia and in Munich, Germany, to promote safe and healthy travel and to facilitate education, service, and research activities in the field of travel medicine. Most useful to the health traveler is the society's searchable database of health travel practitioners.

International Medical Travel Association. Based in Singapore, the International Medical Travel Association (IMTA) and its small but growing membership advocate international patients' rights, quality assurance standards for international hospitals, excellence in continuity of care, and other patient-provider issues. For more information, visit www.intlmta .org.

Beauty from Afar. If you're seeking more specialized information on cosmetic or aesthetic surgery or dental care, author and medical traveler Jeff Schult can fill you in on the main destinations, leading clinics and facilities, and third-party agents. Published in 2006 (Stewart, Tabori & Chang), this 224-page paperback is written in an anecdotal style, providing numerous firsthand accounts that give prospective patients a thorough perspective on the health travel experience.

Medical Tourism in Developing Countries, by Milica Z. Bookman and Karla R. Bookman (Palgrave Macmillan, 2007), explores the international marketplace for medical services and its potential for developing countries. While it's more an academic work than a consumer guide, physicians, administrators, and healthcare officials will find this book's economic perspective and vast bank of data on the industry instructive.

888 STAR.012. Star Hospitals (www .starhospitals.net), a North American healthcare service, operates this toll-free call center staffed entirely by medical professionals. Staff members provide potential clients with information and guidance on member hospitals in India, Singapore, and Thailand.

A couple of magazine articles are worth a trip to your local library or an online search to dig up. If you are considering in vitro fertilization, you need to read "How Far Would You Go to Have a Baby?" by Brian Alexander, which appeared in the May 2005 issue of *Glamour*. On broader topics, Jennifer Wolff's "Passport to Cheaper Health Care?" assesses the pros and cons of medical travel. You'll find it in the October 2007 issue of *Good Housekeeping* or online at www.goodhousekeeping .com.

Web Resources

Medical Nomad. A group of medical professionals, technology geeks, and consultants established www.medical nomad.com in 2004 to bring together an impressive body of information, including specific data on treatments, clinics, physicians, accreditation, and other topics of interest to the health traveler. Medical Nomad's extensive database allows readers to search by procedure, provider, and destination, with clinic and country summaries as well as lay summaries of common treatments.

The Google Guide. While you may not wish to become a wild-eyed expert on the nuances of search engines, a little additional knowledge can greatly enhance your efficiency in narrowing your health travel choices. Consultant and Internet search guru Nancy Blachman (coauthor of the book *How to Do Everything with Google*) has posted a useful online tutorial entitled "The Google Guide." Go to www.googleguide.com, click on "Novice," and you'll find a wealth of information on conducting Internet searches that will greatly improve your online health travel quests. Most of this information applies to other search engines as well, including Yahoo, MSN, and AOL.

RevaHealth.com is a searchable database of healthcare providers. Its unique directory system and powerful search engine allow patients to find detailed information easily. The platform at www.RevaHealth.com also lets patients select providers and talk to them directly for a consultation.

MEDICAL GLOSSARY

Many medical terms are used in this book. The following is a list of the most commonly used terms. For further information, please consult your doctor.

Acute-care. Providing emergency services and general medical and surgical treatment for sudden severe disorders (as compared with long-term care for chronic illness).

Addiction. Occurs when a person has no control over the use of a substance, such as drugs or alcohol. Also includes addictions to food, gambling, and sex.

Aesthetics. A general term for medical treatments and surgical procedures undertaken to improve appearance. Such procedures include (but are not limited to) facelifts, tummy tucks, laser resurfacing of skin, Botox injection, cosmetic dentistry, and others.

Alzheimer's disease. A degenerative disorder of neurons in the brain that disrupts thought, perception, and behavior.

Anesthesia. Loss of physical sensation produced by sedation. Anesthesia may be given as (1) general, which affects the entire body and is accompanied by loss of consciousness; (2) regional, which affects an entire area of the body; and (3) local, which affects a limited part of the body (usually superficial).

Angiography. An x-ray procedure that uses dye injected into the coronary arteries to study circulation in the heart.

Angioplasty. A procedure that uses a tiny balloon on the end of a catheter to widen blocked or constricted arteries in the heart.

Arthroscopy or arthroscopic surgery. The use of a tubelike instrument utilizing fiber optics to examine, treat, or perform surgery on a joint.

Bariatric. Pertaining to the control and treatment of obesity and allied diseases.

Birmingham hip resurfacing (BHR). A metal-on-metal hip replacement system, surgically implanted to replace a hip joint. The BHR is called a resurfacing prosthesis because only the surface of the femoral head (ball) is removed to implant the femoral head-resurfacing component.

Bone densitometry. A method of measuring bone strength, used to diagnose osteoporosis.

Botox. A nonsurgical, physician-administered injection treatment to temporarily reduce moderate to severe wrinkles on the face.

Cardiac. Pertaining to the heart.

Cardiac catheterization. The insertion of a catheter into the arteries of the heart to diagnose heart disease. See also **angiography.**

Cardiothoracic. Pertaining to the heart and the chest.

Cardiovascular. Pertaining to the heart and blood vessels that make up the circulatory system. See also **vascular surgery.**

Cataract. Cloudiness of the lens in the eye, which affects vision. Cataracts, which often occur in older people, can be corrected with surgery to replace the damaged lens with an artificial plastic lens known as an intraocular lens.

Colonoscopy. An examination of the interior of the colon, using a thin, lighted

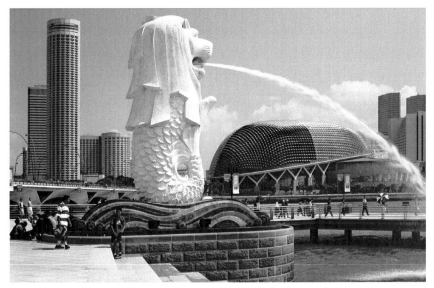

The Merlion is Singapore's national icon

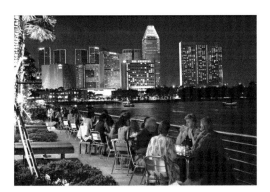

Enjoy the sea breeze and rolling waves against the stunning Singapore skyline while dining at One Fullerton

One Fullerton

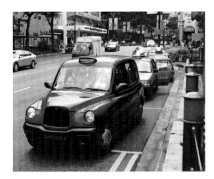

Enjoy hassle-free travel in one of the city's 15,000 air-conditioned cabs

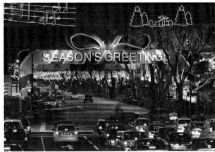

Experience the holidays in the tropics

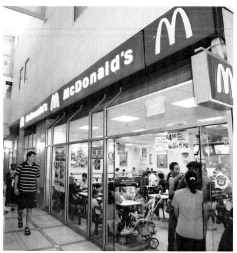

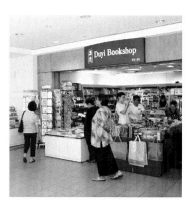

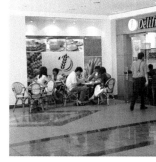

Singapore's hospital lobbies offer a variety of retail stores and familiar eateries

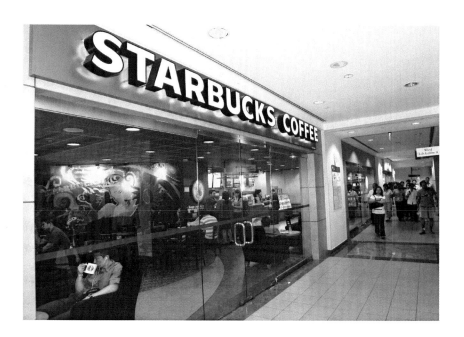

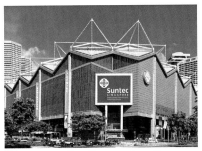

The Suntec City Convention Centre offers 1 million square feet of convention and exhibition space

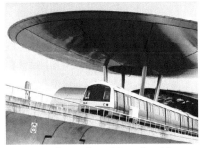

Singapore's modern Mass Rapid Transit system provides convenient, air-conditioned travel throughout the city

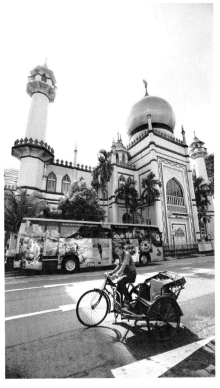

A trishaw tour along Arab Street

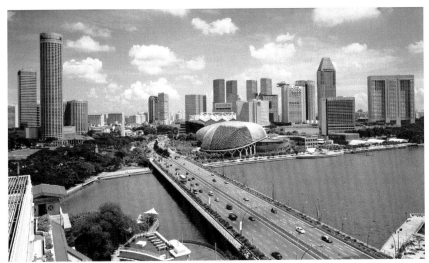

The Singapore River flows through the Central Business District, which is the core of Singapore's commercial and financial activities in the region

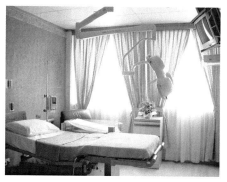

Delivery room at ParkwayHealth's East Shore Hospital

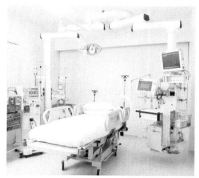

Gleneagles Hospital's Liver Intensive Care Unit

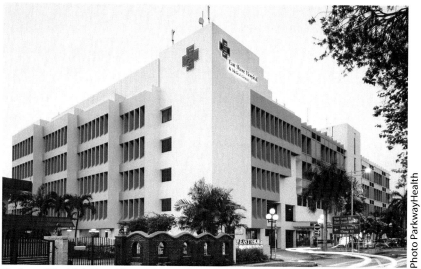

ParkwayHealth's East Shore Hospital

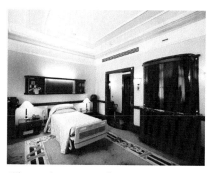

Gleneagles Hospital

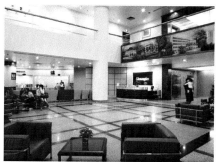

ParkwayHealth's Mount Elizabeth Hospital

tube (a colonoscope) inserted into the rectum.

Computed tomography (CT). Sometimes known as CAT scanning. A noninvasive diagnostic tool that uses x-rays to provide cross-sectional images of the body. Used to detect cancer, determine heart function, and provide images of body organs. May be used in conjunction with **positron emission tomography.**

Coronary artery bypass graft (CABG). Surgical procedure to create alternative paths for blood to flow around obstructions in the coronary arteries, most often using arteries or veins from other parts of the body.

Cosmetic surgery. Plastic surgery undertaken to improve appearance. See also **aesthetics** and **plastic surgery.**

Craniofacial. Pertaining to the head and face.

CyberKnife. A tool for radiosurgery that delivers precise high-dose radiation to a tumor. Can be used for tumors of the pancreas, liver, and lungs.

Diabetes. A chronic disease characterized by abnormally high levels of sugar in the blood.

Discectomy. Removal of all or part of an intervertebral disc (a soft structure that acts as a shock absorber between two bones in the spine).

Electrocardiogram (EKG or ECG). A diagnostic test that measures the heart's electrical activity.

Endocrinology. The branch of medicine that studies hormonal systems and treats disorders that arise when hormones are out of balance.

Endoscope. A slender, tubular optical instrument used as a viewing system for examining an inner part of the body and, with an attached instrument, for performing surgery or detecting tumors.

Extracorporeal shock wave therapy (ESWT). A noninvasive treatment that involves delivery of shock waves to a painful area.

Gamma Knife. A form of radiation therapy that focuses low-dose gamma radiation on a precise target, such as a tumor of the brain or breast.

Gastroenterology. The branch of medicine that studies and treats disorders of the digestive system.

Genetics. The study of inheritance.

Gynecology. The branch of medicine that studies and treats females, especially pertaining to their reproductive system.

Hematology. The study of the nature, function, and diseases of the blood and of blood-forming organs.

Hemopoietic or hematopoietic. Pertaining to the formation of blood.

Hepatitis. Inflammation of the liver caused by a virus or toxin. There are different forms of viral hepatitis. Vaccines are available for hepatitis A and B. There is no vaccine for hepatitis C.

Hepatobiliary. Pertaining to the bile ducts.

Hepatology. The branch of medicine that studies and treats disorders of the liver.

Holter monitor. A wearable electronic device used to obtain a continuous recording of the heart's electrical activity. See **electrocardiogram.**

Immunization. Inoculation with a vaccine to render a person resistant to a disease.

Immunology. The branch of medicine that studies and treats disorders of the body's mechanisms for fighting disease, especially infectious diseases.

Implant. *In dentistry:* a small metal pin placed inside the jawbone to mimic the root of a tooth. Dental implants can be used to help anchor a false tooth, a crown, or a bridge. *In fertility treatment:* to place an embryo in the uterus.

Intensive Care Unit (ICU). The hospital ward in which 24-hour specialized nursing and monitoring are provided for patients who are critically ill or have undergone major surgical procedures.

International Organization for Standardization (ISO). An organization based in Geneva, Switzerland, that approves and accredits the facilities and administrations of hospitals and clinics but not their practices, procedures, or methods.

Intracytoplasmic sperm injection (ICSI). A type of fertility treatment in which a single sperm cell is inserted into an egg using special micromanipulation equipment.

Intrauterine insemination (IUI). Introduction of prepared sperm (either the male partner's or a donor's) into the uterus to improve chances of pregnancy.

In vitro fertilization (IVF). Known as the test-tube baby technique. Eggs are fertilized outside the body, and then embryos are introduced back into the woman's uterus.

Joint Commission International (JCI). The international affiliate accreditation agency of the Joint Commission. JCI inspects and accredits healthcare providers worldwide using US-based standards.

Laparoscope. A thin, lighted tube used to examine and treat tissues and organs inside the abdomen.

LAP-BAND System. An adjustable silicone band inserted laparoscopically around the upper part of the stomach, thereby reducing the stomach's food storage area and promoting weight loss.

LASIK (laser-assisted *in situ* keratomileusis). A laser procedure to reduce dependency on eyeglasses or contact lenses by permanently changing the shape of the cornea, the clear covering of the front of the eye.

Liposuction. The surgical withdrawal of fat from under the skin, using a small incision and suctioning.

Lithotripsy. A procedure that breaks up kidney stones or gallstones using sound waves. Also called extracorporeal shock wave lithotripsy (ESWL).

Magnetic resonance imaging (MRI). A noninvasive diagnostic tool that uses a large magnet, radio waves, and a computer to produce clear images of the interior of the body. Used to diagnose spine and joint problems, heart disease, and cancer.

Mammography. X-ray imaging of the breast for detection of cancer.

Maxillofacial. Pertaining to the jaws and face.

Microsurgical epididymal sperm aspiration (MESA). Obtaining immature sperm cells from the epididymis (which joins the testicle to the vas deferens), in cases where obstruction in the genital tract leads to absence of sperm in the ejaculate. The recovered sperm can be used for **intracytoplasmic sperm injection (ICSI).**

Minimal access surgery. Also called minimally invasive surgery. Any of a variety of approaches used to reduce the trauma of surgery and to speed recovery. These approaches include "keyhole" surgery, endoscopy, arthroscopy, laparoscopy, or the use of small incisions.

Myocardial infarction (MI). Heart attack.

Neonatology. The branch of medicine specializing in the care and treatment of newborns.

Nephrology. The branch of medicine that studies and treats disorders of the kidneys.

Neurology. The branch of medicine that studies and treats disorders of the nervous system, including the brain.

Neuro-oncology. The branch of medicine that studies and treats cancers of the nervous system.

Neuro-ophthalmology. The branch of medicine that studies and treats disorders of the nerves in the eye.

Neurosurgery. Surgery on the brain or other parts of the nervous system.

Obstetrics. The branch of medicine focusing on pregnancy and childbirth.

Oncology. The branch of medicine that studies and treats cancer.

Ophthalmology. The branch of medicine that studies and treats disorders of the eye.

Orthodontics. The branch of dentistry focusing on the prevention and correction of irregular tooth positioning, as by means of braces.

Orthopedics. The branch of medicine that studies and treats diseases and injuries of the bones and joints.

Osteoporosis. Thinning of the bones and reduction in bone mass, which increases the risk of fractures and decreases mobility, especially in the elderly.

Otolaryngology. The branch of medicine that studies and treats ear, nose, and throat disorders.

Pacemaker. An electronic device surgically implanted into a patient's chest to regulate the heartbeat.

Parkinson's disease. A brain disorder that produces movement difficulties, most commonly among the elderly.

Pathology. The branch of medicine focusing on the laboratory-based study of disease in cells and tissues, as opposed to clinical examination of symptoms.

Pediatric. Pertaining to children.

Periodontics. The branch of dentistry focusing on the study and treatment of diseases of the bones, connective tissues, and gums surrounding and supporting the teeth.

Physiotherapy or physical therapy. The treatment or management of physical disability, malfunction, or pain by exercise, massage, hydrotherapy, and other techniques without the use of drugs, surgery, or radiation.

Plastic surgery. The branch of medicine focusing on corrective operations to the face, head, and body to restore function and (sometimes) to improve appearance (also called **cosmetic surgery**).

Polio (poliomyelitis). A paralyzing disease caused by a virus and characterized by inflammation of the motor neurons of the brain stem and spinal cord.

Positron emission tomography (PET). Also known as PET imaging or PET scanning. A diagnostic tool that captures images of the interior of the body by detecting positrons or tiny particles from radioactive material. Used to detect cancer and determine heart function; used most recently as an early clue to Alzheimer's. May be used in conjunction with **computed tomography (CT)**.

Prosthodontics. The branch of dentistry focusing on replacing missing teeth and other oral structures with artificial devices.

Psychiatry. The branch of medicine that studies and treats mental disorders.

Radiofrequency ablation. The use of electrodes to generate heat and destroy abnormal tissue.

Radiology. The branch of medicine focusing on capturing and interpreting images, such as x-rays, CT scans, and MRI scans.

Radiosurgery. The use of ionizing radiation, either from an external source (such as an x-ray machine) or an implant, to destroy cancerous or diseased tissue.

Radiotherapy. Treatment of disease with radiation, especially by selective irradiation with x-rays or other ionizing radiation or by ingestion or implantation of radioisotopes.

Reconstructive surgery. The branch of surgery focusing on the repair or replacement of malformed, injured, or lost organs or tissues of the body, chiefly by the transplant of living tissues.

Rehabilitation. The process of restoring health and improving functioning.

Renal. Pertaining to the kidneys.

Rheumatology. The branch of medicine that studies and treats disorders characterized by pain and stiffness afflicting the extremities or back.

Stem cell. An unspecialized or undifferentiated cell that can become specialized to perform the functions of diverse tissues in the body.

Stent. A tube inserted into a blood vessel or duct to keep it open. Stents are sometimes inserted into narrowed coronary arteries to help keep them open after balloon angioplasty.

Tertiary-care. Providing care of a highly specialized nature.

Testicular epididymal sperm aspiration (TESA). A surgical procedure to obtain sperm from within the testicular tissue.

Transplant. *Organ transplant:* the surgical insertion of an organ from a donor (living or deceased) into a patient to replace an organ that is diseased or malfunctioning; transplants are available for heart, liver, lungs, pancreas, kidney, cornea, and some other organs. *Stem cell transplant:* a procedure in which stem cells are collected from the blood of the patient (autologous) or a matched donor (allogeneic) and then reinserted into the patient to rebuild the immune system. *Bone marrow transplant:* a procedure that places healthy bone marrow from the patient (autograft) or a donor (allograft) into a patient whose bone marrow is damaged or malfunctioning.

Typhoid. An infectious, potentially fatal intestinal disease caused by bacteria and usually transmitted in food or water.

Ultrasound. The use of high-frequency sound waves in therapy or diagnostics, as in the deep-heat treatment of a joint or in the imaging of internal structures.

Urology. The branch of medicine that studies and treats urinary tract infections (UTIs) and other disorders of the urinary system.

Vascular surgery. The branch of medicine focusing on the diagnosis and surgical treatment of disorders of the blood vessels, excluding the heart, lungs, and brain.

Wellness. An area of preventive medicine that promotes health and well-being though various means, such as diet, exercise, yoga, tai chi, social support, and more.

X-rays. A form of electromagnetic radiation, similar to light but of shorter wavelength, which can penetrate solids; used for imaging solid structures inside the body.

INDEX

Hospital names and specialist groups are in **bold**. Main treatment categories are indexed in *italics*; specific treatments may be found in the text.

ABOUT THE AUTHOR

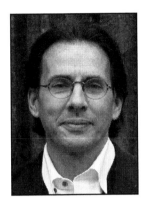

As President of Healthy Travel Media, **Josef Woodman** has spent more than three years touring 100 medical facilities in 14 countries, researching contemporary medical tourism. As co-founder of MyDailyHealth and Ventana Communications, Woodman's pioneering background in health, wellness, and Web technology has allowed him to compile a wealth of information about global health travel, telemedicine, and new developments in consumer and institutional medical care. Woodman has lectured at the UCLA School of Public Health and Harvard Medical School and has conducted seminars and workshops in a dozen countries. He serves on the Advisory Board of the Global Healthcare Summit and as Program Co-Chairman of the Global Healthcare Congress. Woodman has emerged as an outspoken advocate of global consumer healthcare and medical travel.

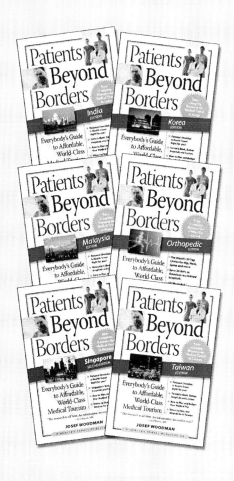